MoneyWise Weight Loss

The Faith-based Plan for Building a Better
Body on a Budget

Kimberly Floyd

Wellspring Omnimedia

Disclaimer

The information in this guide should be considered as general information only and should not be used to diagnose medical conditions. This guide is sold with the understanding that neither the publisher nor author is engaged in rendering medical advice. Please see your health care provider for diagnosis and treatment of any medical concerns, and before implementing any diet, exercise or other lifestyle changes.

Dedication

I dedicate this book to all those who struggle with their weight, particularly those who might be weary in the journey right now.

Here's a little encouragement for you:

> You may say "I can't,"
> But you know that God can.
> If His spirit is in you,
> Then you know you can.
> So now, ask yourself "Will I?"

Today, say "I will!" Heaven knows you are worth it!

Table of Contents

Introduction

MY STORY

My body and I had been enemies for as long as I could remember. It finally became my friend in my late thirties, and that was only after a painful wake-up call. I now see my body as God's temple, the most precious gift He has given me. The joy I feel now has made it worth every step it took for me to get here.

I was once 240 lbs and a size 22. Following his usual lecture about my need to lose weight, my former gynecologist added something new. In frustration, he said that the effect my obesity was having on my heart was like asking an engine designed for a Volkswagen to haul the weight of a Mack truck.

Shaken by his blunt words, I sat down in my car and cried. But that wasn't enough to motivate a change. Instead, I went home and comforted myself the only way I thought I knew how: by eating the coconut cake in my refrigerator—the entire cake.

My problem wasn't lack of knowledge about health. After all, I was a registered nurse at the time and knew about nutrition and exercise. The problem was that I didn't *want* to do it. I enjoyed eating and it was the only self-nurturing method for which I made time. Food made me feel loved and special. It was the faulty way I chose to deal with the stress in my life.

Because I worked long hours, I had little energy to do much when I arrived home except watch television. It seemed easier to grab fast food instead of preparing meals for myself. And exercising? Forget about it!

Besides, nearly everyone around me was overweight including my friends and fellow nurses. Each time I announced my ambition to lose the weight for good, they would nod their heads with amused looks that seemed to say "Yeah, right."

Unfortunately, they knew me all too well.

I had dieted and lost the weight many times, but it always crept back—and then some. This was in spite of spending thousands of dollars on weight loss programs, exercise equipment, and workout regimens. But after the wake-up call, I made a firm decision to lose the weight the right way and it never came back. You see,

I finally learned to *stop putting my body's care last on my priority list.*

Two years after the doctor's "Mack truck" comment, I began having problems with my blood pressure. I have a strong history of high blood pressure in my family. In fact, my grandmother died from a stroke at the age of 47. Family pictures show that she was obviously overweight. Six months after her death, my great-grandmother also died from a stroke. My mother, aunt, and cousins all had high blood pressure and it appeared I was next on the hypertension hit list.

My general physician put me on pills to manage my condition, but these only made me feel worse. One night, I fell asleep on the sofa while watching television. Earlier, I had set the alarm clock in my bedroom and was startled awake by the sound of it. As I jumped up from the sofa to run and turn it off, an excruciating pain slammed into my chest.

This pain was like nothing I had ever felt before. It was as if someone had reached inside of my ribcage, grabbed my heart, and gave it a brutal squeeze. The pain lasted only a second but it terrified me.

While I stood there, hand over my heart and afraid to take another step, I saw the truth of what I had been doing to my body with poor health habits. My little "Volkswagen engine" heart was at last rebelling against the extra weight I had forced it to carry.

It was also during that moment that I heard God's voice: "It is not supposed to be this way." I chose right then to believe Him and how my life changed! Later that week, I had an appointment with the doctor and I wrote on the back of the appointment card: *Today is the day I turn my life around.*

Those events occurred several years ago. Since then, I have shed 85 pounds and 14 dress sizes (from a size 22 to size 8). Just before I made the decision to lose weight, I had taken a great class about managing money from a biblical perspective. At the time, I had an alarming $19,000 worth of credit card debt. I set a goal to get out of debt in 5 years yet God graciously provided a means to pay it off in just 3 years, 11 months. I discovered the truth that when the student is ready, the teacher appears!

I applied the same principles I had used to gain control of my financial life to take control of my physical body. I hope to pass the same principles on to you in this book. I now teach them in my *Take Back Your Temple* seminars, which are designed to help others experience the freedom of building healthy lifestyles.

I truly believe that when you value something, you take care of it. You are *valuable*. May this book give you a new appreciation for your body, and what God designed it to do. I hope you will also take the principles to heart and use them to transform your body, health, finances, and ultimately your life. Ideally you will pass them on to others so they too can experience the abundant life that is available to all who are willing to receive it.

REVERSING THE OBESITY TREND

This book grew out of a series of speeches I had given at churches in the Atlanta area. Many times after my talks, I was approached by other women and men who told me about their own struggles with weight. I couldn't help but notice the desperation behind each of their stories. I recognized it because I had felt the same way, hoping all the time that I would find a way out of the prison my body had become. I have discovered that there are millions in the same situation.

While rates of overweight have risen among Americans in general, the percentages are particularly high among certain minority groups. According to the American Obesity Association, over 69% of African Americans and 73.4% of Hispanics are overweight. High percentages of these populations are also classified as severely overweight (obese).

Just take a look at some statistics from the *Healthwatch* organization about how obesity-related illnesses are affecting African American women specifically. This group is bearing the brunt of such illnesses:

- Death rates from cardiovascular disease are 35% higher for African-American women than for white women

- Hypertension occurs at a rate of 34.2% in African-American females compared to 19.3% of white females

- Diabetes occurs at a rate of 16 to 26% in Hispanic and African-Americans, aged 45–74, compared to 12% in whites of the same age group

To see these statistics played out, you need not look very far. Just consider your family, fellow church members, co-workers, and friends. The chances are that you associate frequently with someone who is suffering from these diseases.

Why are these illnesses becoming rampant? Our society today actually fosters fat storage. It has become all too easy to eat a so-called 'poor folks diet.' These diets feature foods that are high in fat and sugar. They are cheap and fill you up, but provide little nutritional value to the body. Worst of all these foods provide an extraordinary number of calories (energy units) in even small servings, so it doesn't take much of them to exceed the body's needs.

List: favorite foods

It is also easy to avoid exercise. Many of us have desk jobs that require us to exercise our minds, but not our bodies. We drive our cars almost everywhere, take escalators, use riding lawnmowers, and try to find the closest parking space at the shopping center.

What you do to exercise.

To relax, we like to watch television, read, and play cards or board games. Our children play video games. There was a time when kids would play actively outside for hours; now parents can hardly get them *out* of the house. We have become an overly sedentary society.

What you do to relax

The rates of obesity among children are increasing just as fast as those for adults. Not only that, but even young children are starting to show signs of heart disease and diabetes. At an age when they should be carefree, many children are being burdened by obesity-related illnesses and the discomfort that goes along with them.

While surfing the Internet recently, I came upon a Web site that publicized the emotional pain which often accompanies obesity. The Web site contained letters from people who were battling the condition—and losing. The letters broke my heart. Can you imagine what it would be like trying to live a victorious life under these conditions?

checklist

- "I'm tired all the time...."
- "I've lost my joy over the years...."
- "I feel guilty for letting myself get so big...."
- "I am filled with depression and hopelessness...."
- "I don't want my children to have to go through this...."

While I cannot relate to these statements anymore, there was a time when I could sympathize with many of them.

I wrote this book in an effort to prevent you from becoming (or staying) part of the obesity statistics. Even more than that, I want to help you end weight as an issue in your life once and for all. We sometimes become so comfortable in our struggles with weight that they start to feel normal, especially if the people around us are in the same shape.

While God made us in all shapes and sizes, obesity is *not* a natural condition. It doesn't take a genius to figure out that taking in more food than the body needs plus an inactive lifestyle will make us overweight. If the habits continue long enough we will eventually become obese. We must reverse the trend by eating foods that build healthy bodies and by moving our temples as God designed. We may not be able to eat a perfect diet or run a marathon, but we can do *better* than we are doing now. All it takes is for us to be willing to pursue good health, one small step at a time. We can start right where we are and have fun doing it!

Make a decision to take this journey for the sake of your friends, neighbors, coworkers, spouses and for your children. Most importantly, do it for yourself because you can only give the best of yourself to others when you are strong, healthy, and vibrant.

I believe God's desire is for you to care for yourself so you can be fit to care for others. You honor Him when you are good to your body. By taking care of yourself, you demonstrate good stewardship of this wonderful gift He has given you. Eating a healthy diet and getting regular physical activity is one of the best ways to affirm your worth and value.

God himself described your body as a temple, a dwelling that is beautiful, sacred, precious, and valuable. But unlike an actual temple made of stone or brick, your body isn't stable. It is dynamic, constantly changing in response to the food you eat and the movement you make. With your daily choices, you promote health or sickness in your body. God's desire is for you to choose wisely.

Your first important choice is to love your body, respect it, and appreciate its worth. According to a *Wired* magazine article, the human body is worth more than $45 million if you consider the value of your tissues, fluids, organs, and germ antibodies. So start thinking of yourself as a *$45 million dollar baby*! Value your body exactly the way it is now while you are losing weight and rebuilding your health, not just when you achieve your goal. This will keep you motivated. God loves you unconditionally and cares for you no matter what size you are. So should *you.*

HOW TO USE THIS BOOK

The title *MoneyWise Weight Loss* speaks to two important points. The first is to encourage you to be *wise* and stop spending your money on quick weight loss fixes, like extreme diets, pills, potions, and the like. After years of trying these methods myself, the only thing that ultimately ended up lighter was my wallet. My advice to you is to save your money and get healthy the lasting, scriptural way.

Give me all your money, and then we'll go home.

Everything worth achieving takes time. Changing your body does too. If you want your changes to last (which is the key), then you need to make sure that you are making them in a way that builds your health up rather than tears it down as quick fixes tend to do. You also want to build fun into the process, which is the missing ingredient in many health programs.

The second point is that you can save *money* on certain foods that will help you lose weight. That is what distinguishes this book from any other on the market. Many diets plans are expensive, providing tasty recipes but with ingredients that put a serious dent in your wallet.

MoneyWise Weight Loss recognizes that most of us don't have access to unlimited funds. It respects the fact that you may be budget conscious and so provides suggestions for meals, snacks, and recipes that use economical ingredients that are easily obtainable.

Another of the book's key features is a checklist of tips at the end of each chapter. You'll select the ones that will work best for your life. At the end of the book, you will compile the small steps into a complete roadmap for losing weight that is customized for you.

The following is some additional information about how the book is structured:

- Part 1: *Laying the foundation* helps you establish your vision for the health goals you want to accomplish. You will also learn about the spiritual and mental aspects of losing weight, which will keep you on target with your goal.

- Part 2: *Building a Better Body* gives you the tools and materials you need to start creating your health vision, one small step at a time. You'll learn about simple methods to prevent overeating and how to save money on healthy food. Furthermore, you'll discover how to fix your plate to lose weight with every bite, and increase your energy and strength by moving your body creatively.

- Part 3: *Finishing Touches* answers the question, "What do I do after achieving my ideal weight?" It provides a plan for maintenance to ensure that you continue to pursue good health long after you have read the last page.

THE PROMISE OF THIS BOOK

I want you to take away the following message by the time you finish this book: Caring for your body is ultimately about wise stewardship, not about size. It is not important whether your weight is higher than society's "ideal." What matters is that you eat and exercise in a consistently healthful way. God can give you the power to make your health vision a reality, but you must make it happen.

It's not too late. All you have to do is decide that you are willing to take the steps. Come on, it's the least you can do as a $45 million dollar baby. I promise you no regrets! Don't wait to start looking your best and feeling your finest. There's no better day to start than *today*!

Part 1

Laying the Foundation

Chapter 1: Making the Trade

"A vision is not just a picture of what could be; it is an appeal to our better selves, a call to become something more."

—Rosabeth Moss Kanter, Speaker and Consultant

Is this your first time attempting to lose weight? If you are like most people reading this book, it's not your first, your second, or even your fifth attempt. As you read in the introduction, this author tried losing weight dozens of times before getting it right. The last time was different because *I* was different: I associated literal pain in my chest with my former habits and was determined to trade them in for ones that would give me better results. I wanted to live a life of energy, vitality, and joy, which I was sorely lacking at the time.

Have you taken time to think of compelling reasons for wanting to lose weight? Until you come to realize that you are trading up to a better way of *daily* life by making positive health changes, then you probably won't stick with it long-term. In this chapter, I will share with you how to clarify your reasons and create a strong vision of vibrant health. You will also find the one tool that you need to transform your vision from dream to reality: a viable plan.

The Bible tells us that we should *write* the vision and make it plain. Studies show that our commitment to goals is much stronger when we write them down than just trying to rely on memory. It is all too easy to forget goals when the realities and demands of life intrude and divert our attention.

Since you will be working on renovating your temple, it may help to visualize this process like you would any other building project. Just as a person wouldn't attempt to build or renovate a house without a plan, so you should never attempt your health transformation without one. With a plan, your chances of success increase greatly.

A good life-changing plan will answer the following questions:

- What is my situation now?
- What do I want it to be?
- What am I willing to do to change the situation?
- What resources do I have that can help me?

Let's take a look at each of these elements so you can start the planning process.

DEFINE YOUR CURRENT SITUATION

Just as an architect surveys the land on which she wants to build, so you must survey your own "territory." You need to clearly state what you want to alter and start identifying any obstacles that could potentially interfere.

This step is critical. Suppose our architect fails to perform a site analysis and builds her house anyway, only to see it crumble before her eyes because she built it on quicksand? Taking time to define your current situation and foreseeing potential roadblocks brings matters out into the open so that you can prepare to deal with them.

So what kind of questions can assist you in defining your current situation? You may begin by answering the following questions:

What is my current weight and height or clothing size?

_____

_____

_____

_____

What benefits do I receive by **not** changing?

_____

_____

_____

_____

_____

What has prevented me from changing before now?

_____

_____

_____

_____

Were you surprised by those last two questions? Part of your survey is taking an honest look at what you have to lose or gain by shedding pounds. Many times, we consider the benefits of losing weight but fail to uncover any perceived "downsides." However, it is those possible pitfalls that have the potential to trip you up.

In some people's minds, there are benefits to remaining overweight and to savoring its associated poor nutrition habits and low physical activity. These so-called "benefits" can deceive you and keep you from giving it your best effort. Do not let such thoughts hinder you from reaching your ideal weight and cause you to sabotage yourself unconsciously.

For example, a woman named Cindy wanted to lose a significant amount of weight, but thought that she had the following "benefits" of remaining overweight:

- I'm afraid of men. By remaining severely overweight, I feel I'm invisible to them so I don't have to worry about receiving attention from them.

- I don't have to deal with change. I can just continue my normal pattern of working, preparing food, eating, watching television, and sleeping.

- I can continue to use food to mask any feelings I don't want to deal with, like anger towards my mother for her verbal abuse when I was a child.

- I can eat exactly what I want, how much I want, when I want, and I don't have to exercise.

- I don't have to worry about spending money to look fashionable on new clothes (unless I continue to gain weight and then I'd have to spend money for larger sizes).

- I don't have to deal with questions from friends or family, asking "Are you on a diet...again?"

- I don't have to deal with the uncomfortable feelings of controlling my eating when everyone else around me is eating unhealthy food and pigging out.

Are there any statements with which you can identify after reading Cindy's list? Take a look at the way you currently spend your time. Examine the relationships you have with your friends and family. Consider how things might change if you did slim down. What do you think will likely happen?

Set your timer for 5 minutes. Quickly complete the right side of the chart that follows (Reasons to stay the same). Write the first things that come to your mind.

Reasons to lose weight (Gains)	Reasons to stay the same (Losses)

How did listing your losses make you feel? Were you sad, frustrated, or scared? Again, the information is important to have because it may point to potential obstacles. If this exercise seemed a little depressing, don't worry. We are about to look on the bright side.

DEFINE YOUR FUTURE SITUATION

Now you will have an opportunity to precisely state your future health goal. You must be very specific and have a timeframe assigned to it. For example "In two months, I will wear a size 10 dress size." Write down a target date when you want to look and feel your best. If it helps, close your eyes and see yourself having achieved your goal. What are you doing? Who are you with? What are you wearing? How do you feel? Make your vision as vivid as possible.

Remember the saying "If you can't see it, you can't be it." Write down your goal and health vision now.

_____

_____

_____

_____

_____

_____

Great job! Now that you have recorded your goal and vision, let's return to the chart on which you previously worked. This time, complete the *left* side of the chart (Reasons to lose weight). Set your timer for 5 minutes and go!

Now that both sides are filled in, take a good look at the chart. If your reasons to stay the same are longer than your reasons to lose weight or if you find yourself defending your overweight state, then you may sabotage your efforts to lose weight. Are you prepared to endure the misery of such an outcome? God wants so much more for you!

You see, you'll need convincing reasons to begin and continue this project. Some days will be easy, but others will be challenging. God will give you the ability to focus on the benefits you will gain to keep you going during the tough times. Without seeking His guidance, your flesh will cause you to give up with the slightest opposition from others or with the first temptation. You need not let this happen. So, please take another five minutes to make additions to your "gains" column. As you write, think about the fun that you will have while achieving your goal. Be certain to make your reasons real and meaningful to you.

If you need help coming up with additional benefits of becoming trim, then take a look at the benefits list that Cindy created to encourage herself to lose weight and adopt positive health habits:

- I can gain peace about my health habits. I don't have peace about them right now because I know what I should do, but don't do it.

- I want to deal with my feelings head on. I want to stop using food as a substitute for God.

- I want to be in control of myself and my eating. Right now, I feel out of control.

- I want to be free to shop for clothes at *any* store, not just limited to large lady stores or departments.

- I want to be a health inspiration to my friends and family with my testimony of God's faithfulness during the weight loss.

- I want to have stable moods; right now they are all over the place.

- I want to stop getting intoxicated with sugar.

- I want to be able to run and climb stairs without getting out of breath.

- I want to feel pleased to know I am treating myself well in all areas.

- I want to look in the mirror and like what I see. All over.

- I want to be sexually confident when I marry, to be able to make love with the lights on.

- I want to age well and maintain my mobility. I want to have a sharp mind and fit body.

- I want to be able to go to the movies or to sporting events without worrying about whether I will fit into the seats.

- I want to stay healthy for life and I know that nutrition and exercise are a major part of that.

- I spend a lot of money on fast food and eating out. I want to save and invest that money instead.

- I want to have energy I need to accomplish my goals and to fulfill my God-given purpose.

Here is another exercise that should help you strengthen your positive reasons for starting. If you lost weight, what would be the best outcome for you and others because of it? For example, here is a possible list of best case scenarios:

- If you lost weight and developed good health habits, you could pass those on to your children and they would be healthier.

- Your children would teach your grandchildren good health habits and that would continue throughout the generations.

- Because the family's health habits have improved, its members may not have to suffer from diabetes, high blood pressure, and strokes as the generations before them.

- When you reach your ideal weight, you will likely inspire friends to do the same.

- Your friends will in turn teach their children good health habits.

- Your friends' children will then teach their own children to live healthfully and will pass them on to their descendants.

This was merely a brief list. Your choosing to become your ideal weight could also affect your neighbors, coworkers, fellow church or club members in a positive way. It will also likely give you the energy you need to pursue new interests, relationships, or even an exciting career. And who knows where any of this could lead?

Please take 10 minutes to complete the list that follows. Dream big and don't judge. Again, write the first answers that enter your mind. You can always add more or change them later.

If I achieved my ideal weight, what would be the best outcome for me and for others in my circle of influence?

1._____

2._____

3. _____

4. _____

5._____

6. _____

7. _____

8. _____

9. _____

10. _____

It is astonishing when you begin to realize how much your life and the choices you make affect others. You must never forget this is because you truly have God's power to make a positive impact on those around you. That will in turn affect these people and impact those whom they contact.

What conclusions did you draw? Do you think you are ready to start? If you have found that you don't have enough reasons to begin, then take the matter to God prayerfully and ask Him to reveal to you reasons to work on this issue. When you are able to record enough positive reasons to begin so that they overtake the losses column, rejoice! Then you are ready to embark upon the journey to true victory.

WHAT I'M WILLING TO DO

In this part of your plan, you will need to be honest about what you are willing to do to accomplish your health goal. At this stage, you consider your level of motivation, potential obstacles (including any mental ones like those listed in the 'losses' column completed earlier) and your decisive plan for dealing with them.

For example, let's suppose that one of the listed losses was that you are accustomed to going out with a girlfriend every Friday night for coffee and a rich dessert. You enjoy the time you spend with her and are afraid that you will have to sacrifice that if you want to lose weight. What are you willing to do to deal with this obstacle?

After thinking about it, you realize that the time spent with your friend isn't the problem; it's the coffee and rich dessert that come with it. So you start thinking of ways that you could still spend time with your friend but minus the coffee and dessert.

The solution that you are willing to implement might include asking your friend if you can instead meet her on a local walking trail to catch up; you might ask her if you can order one dessert and split it with her; or you could order a sorbet or fruit parfait from the menu instead of the 'Death by Chocolate' dessert that you usually order. No, you don't have to say goodbye to 'Death by Chocolate' forever but you should not have it every week if you want to achieve your weight loss goal in the timeframe you have set. Instead, you might save it for special occasions.

I hope you see now that identifying obstacles and creating a plan to deal with them is crucial. Take a moment to think about obstacles you might face in reducing your size and determine what you are willing to do to overcome the barriers.

Set your timer for 15 minutes and complete the
table.

Potential obstacle to losing weight	My solution for overcoming this obstacle

DETERMINE YOUR RESOURCES

Now that you have written down your obstacles
and a plan for dealing with them you will need to take
inventory of the resources available to help you succeed.
Conducting the inventory ensures that you are taking full
advantage of every source of help at your disposal.

Remember at the beginning of the chapter when I
asked you whether this was your first time attempting to
lose weight? If you have attempted to shed pounds

multiple times, then you have one of the best resources available: experience. You have some idea of what has worked well for you in the past and what hasn't. You already paid for that experience so you might as well cash it in by walking in the wisdom gleaned!

Here are some other resources you have:

- God
- Time
- Other people
- Creativity
- Money

You might look at the list and think that you have limited amounts of both time and money. While that may be true, you also have creativity, which helps you create solutions to obstacles related to limited time and money.

Another good resource that you hopefully have is the support of other people. The old saying that 'no man (or woman) is an island' is true; you need support to succeed with your efforts long term.

In your own relationships, do you have someone who can encourage you in your weight/financial quest? Do you have someone who knows about good nutrition whose knowledge you can apply? One of the best resources possible is someone who has already achieved the goals that you want to reach—and did so in a healthy way. That person can serve as a role model and/or accountability partner. We will discuss this concept more later in the book.

Last and most importantly, you have God as a resource if you are willing to seek the One who created you and knows you best. Even if no one else is in your corner, then God is the ultimate support system! You are promised that you can do all things through Christ who strengthens you. Be assured by this promise boldly and begin walking as if you believe it.

If you are reluctant to enlist God's help with your weight issues due to fear of failure or sacrifice remember that such fear is not of Him. "God did not give you a spirit of fear but of power, love, and a sound mind (2 Timothy 1:7)." When you truly grasp that your Creator does not want your body to be a burden to you or for you to live a life consumed by fear, then you will be on your way to becoming the person that He designed you to be.

Remember the health vision you wrote down earlier? If you felt good thinking about it and are passionate about seeing it come to fruition then you might say that you are *enthusiastic* about your vision. The word *enthusiastic* actually means *inspiration from God*.

So if God has given you this vision of better health and quality of life, then it will come to pass. But your cooperation is critical; without consistent effort toward achieving the vision, it will die and you will not secure the best God has to offer you. Make no mistake about it; this is serious business.

One way to keep your vision alive is to keep it in front of your eyes. Write your vision as a short statement. Add words like "fun," "easy," and "love" to this sentence. Write the statement as if you have already achieved your goal. Here is an example: "It is <u>fun</u> being a size 10 and it is <u>easy</u> taking care of myself every day." Your brain is drawn to activities that are fun and easy!

I recommend copying your vision on large index cards as recommended in Earl Nightingale's audio program and book, *The Strangest Secret*. Below that, write the following scripture:

"Ask, and it will be given to you; seek, and you will find; knock, and it will be opened to you."

- Matthew 7:7

Tape the cards on your bathroom mirror, refrigerator, computer, or any place where you are likely to see them. Read them out loud eight times a day with enthusiasm and power. When you do this, you speak life into your vision.

Pay attention to your thoughts. Whenever you have negative, doubting thoughts related to your vision, replace them with thoughts that are supportive and faith filled. Do this for the next 30 days--if you have a negative thought about your vision then just start over as if it were day one. Your goal is to make it through an entire 30-day stretch with thoughts that are 100% supportive.

Also, see the vision coming to pass. For five minutes twice a day, close your eyes and see yourself at your ideal size. Feel pleasure from it. While you are visualizing, see yourself eating healthy and enjoying it; see yourself living a fun, active life.

These activities will keep you focused. When you do them, your enthusiasm will grow, you will work through your plan, and your vision will unfold right before your eyes.

Small Steps Action Plan - Making the Trade

Place a checkmark next to the following actions you are willing to take to see your health vision come to pass.

Review this list once a week to be sure you are following through on your decision.

❑ Write down what my current situation is (current weight/size).

❑ Record what I want my future situation to be (future weight/size).

❑ Complete the gain/loss table regarding losing weight and make sure my gains list is longer than the losses.

❑ Write down my health vision in detail.

❑ Write down the best possible outcomes for my weight loss.

❑ Write down obstacles I could face in losing weight and my plan for overcoming them.

❑ Speak life into my health vision by reading it out loud twice a day from the index cards as recommended.

❑ Visualize twice a day my health vision coming to pass.

❑ Pray for strength often.

Chapter 2: Knowing Your True Source

"Whether fear or faith prevails depends on the commander we are saluting."

–Beth Moore, Author and Bible Teacher

I am fully convinced that increasing my knowledge of God was the primary reason for success in taking back my temple. The turning point came when I realized that I had begun thinking more about God during the day than about food.

In my previous attempts at weight loss, food was a stubborn obsession: I obsessed over amounts or I thought about the food I *couldn't* have. This pattern of thinking was a stronghold in my mind. Whenever I felt a negative emotion, my first thought was to run to food to make myself feel better.

To see what a powerful stronghold food can be, imagine how some oft-quoted bible verses would sound if we replaced God/Lord with food:

- "The joy of <u>food</u> is my strength."
- "<u>Food</u> heals the brokenhearted and binds up their wounds."

- "Be strong and let your heart take courage, all you who hope in <u>food</u>."
- "Trust in <u>food</u> with all your heart and do not lean on your own understanding."
- "The righteous man will be glad in <u>food</u> and will take refuge in <u>it</u>; and all the upright in heart will glory."

Those statements might seem funny, yet many of us live as if we believe them. I know I did. Food is not supposed to be a god in your life, but that is what it became in mine.

Overeating can have little to do with food; sometimes we overeat because the food is tasty or because it is simply there. But other times, it stems from a desire to fill up empty parts of ourselves, a desire to comfort ourselves and avoid dealing with past hurts, disappointments, and pain. However, food can never solve emotional issues; only God can.

Scientific research states that when we are attempting to change habits, we must replace them with new ones. If we don't, a vacuum is created where the old habits used to be. Nature hates a vacuum. If we haven't already chosen good habits to fill the space, then bad ones are free to enter and take up residence.

The habits I will discuss in this chapter can help you strengthen yourself spiritually so that God can assume His rightful place in your mind: First. I call these habits $P\ W^2$: prayer, praise, worship, and word.

Together, they will help you increase your levels of self control, which is the key to weight loss success.

PRAYER

I always think of prayer as being similar to accessing a Global Positioning System (GPS). The GPS system is a series of satellites that can pinpoint your location from anywhere on earth as long as you have a GPS receiver and a clear view of the sky. Many expensive cars have GPS systems, which help their owners navigate from their current location to their ultimate destination.

With a strong prayer life, you increase your sensitivity to God's voice. When you follow His lead, you won't lose your way to your destination of better health!

A University of Arizona study showed that people who engaged in regular spiritual practices like prayer had significantly lower levels of the stress hormone *cortisol*. Cortisol has been linked to the body's mechanisms for fat storage, particularly belly fat. When cortisol levels are lowered, stress-related abdominal fat storage is lowered.

Consider the following additional benefits of a strong prayer life:

- You will gain insight into God's character
- You will learn about God's will for your life as He reveals it
- You will gain strength to conquer your health challenges
- You will learn how to trust in God, which will reduce your stress level

For those of you who are thinking, "I would love to have a mighty prayer life, but I don't know how to pray" then you are about to learn. A pattern for effective prayer is outlined in Matthew 6:9. Jesus first proclaims God as His Father. Similarly, we should begin our prayer life by claiming God as our father.

I must admit that I formerly had problems seeing God as my Father. I believe this was because the idea of calling someone "father" or "daddy" was foreign to me. My earthly father had abandoned my family, so I had no concept of receiving unconditional love from a father.

Many women (particularly minority women) grew up without fathers in the home, either through physical absence or through emotional absence. You can begin allowing God to heal this part of your life by claiming Him as yours, just as Jesus did. Your Father's name is to be hallowed, which means deserving of reverence, respect, and honor. You can't have a better Father than that!

Next, we ask God to supply our needs on a daily basis, not only our physical needs, but also our spiritual and emotional ones. Since God knows everything, He is aware of our needs even before we ask. But in taking the step to ask Him, we acknowledge that all that we receive comes from Him. Part of asking for provision is asking God to give you wisdom to choose food that will bring strength and vitality to your body. Pray that He will guide you on the correct amounts that you should eat to be sustained.

Forgiveness is the next thing that we ask for in prayer. In the Lord's Prayer Jesus asked God to "forgive our debts" *as* we forgive others for their debts to us. This means that God can only forgive our sins if we readily forgive others theirs. Holding unforgiveness in your heart can be a major contributor to your weight problem because you may overeat to mask the pain from the negative emotions you feel. Forgiveness allows you to release those negative emotions so that you can free yourself from that stronghold and move on with your life.

The last thing that we request in prayer is *protection*. Most martial artists know that the best way to deal with a conflict is to avoid getting into one in the first place.

In your health journey, you've probably already discovered that there are certain foods with which you have a problem: When you eat them, you have a tendency to overindulge. So the most effective way is to avoid them altogether. Don't put yourself at risk by keeping temptations directly in front of you because this will set the stage for your eventual downfall.

When you ask God for protection and to order your steps away from temptation, pay attention to His direction and obey. For example, if you always pass a donut shop on the way to work and you are accustomed to going inside for breakfast, He may help you remember an alternate route to work that avoids the area. Or He may help you shift your focus so that you don't notice the donut shop at all. By obeying these promptings you will find that the confidence in your ability to fulfill your vision will soar and you will achieve it a lot faster.

My recommendation is to begin your day with prayer. In this way, you say to God: "Here I am; do with me as You will." You need God's power and wisdom to help you handle daily conflicts, in particular those related to caring for your body so you might as well start your day off right!

The length of time that you pray depends on how much of God's power you want demonstrated in your life. I recommend a goal of 15 minutes in the morning to start, which is over five times the U.S. average. As your prayer life increases, so will your confidence.

Don't think of this time as a legalistic rule you must follow; some days you may speak with God for less than 15 minutes and some days more. The point is to acknowledge that you can't do this alone. Humbling yourself and asking for God's assistance gives you power to honor Him in everything that you do that day, including the way that you eat.

PRAISE

There is no better way to cultivate joy than to praise God consistently for what He has done in our lives. The bible tells us that we should put on the garment of praise for a spirit of heaviness. We must make a conscious effort to do it since it is not natural for us.

Praise shifts our focus from the negatives in our lives toward the positives. It allows us to enjoy what we have more and brings peace and contentment. With a praise perspective, we are less likely to stress over minor annoyances. Since many of us tend to overeat when we are stressed or anxious, we may be less likely to do so if we engage in regular praise. We can also endure challenges more gracefully.

Many of us carry around burdens related to unwise actions in our past. Even though you may have returned to the right path, you often still have to deal with the consequences of these actions…at least for a while.

For example, you will experience the consequences of poor health habits by the excess weight you carry, at least until your body remakes itself from your newer, healthier habits. However, realize that your current body is only a snapshot from your past—it's the result of thousands of choices you made back then. The choices you make today can create a better body. You've already started making better choices just by buying this book!

So I recommend that your first act of praise be that God has given you a vision of health and the means to accomplish it. Your goal today is to find six more things for which to praise God.

In Psalm 119:164, the Psalmist says that he will praise the Lord seven times a day because of His righteous judgments. I recommend that you do the same! Start an outrageous praise journal. In a blank book or journal designed for the purpose, simply record seven things each day for 31 days for which you want to praise God.

Your notebook should be small enough for you to carry around with you so that you can jot down your praise right on the spot. We tend to forget these things easily! As you begin to pay attention to what is right in your life instead of what is wrong, you will find much more than seven things per day for which to praise Him.

By the end of the 31 days, you should have a minimum of 217 things for which you are grateful to God. If you like, you can continue the journal on and on! I believe praise is a simple way to practice His presence. Every time you praise Him, you can be sure that He is close by and is listening.

Mentally note your attitude before the 31 days of outrageous praise compared to your attitude afterwards.

You will have more energy and joy, actually wanting to do things that preserve your health. Prove it for yourself.

WORSHIP

Praise and worship are often used in the same sentence as if having identical meanings, but they are different. With praise, we show gratitude to God for what He has done for us; with worship, we show reverence to God for who He *is*.

God has given us a tremendous gift in worship. He has removed the boundaries and barriers that were previously in place in the Old Testament. Since Jesus paid the price, we have free access to God. In giving us the kind of worship that is not restricted by place or time, He has given us the opportunity to experience "heaven on earth." For a while, we can escape the cares of this world and experience oneness in spirit with Him. When we are spiritual refreshed, we are also less likely to engage in destructive health behaviors in a misguided attempt to fill ourselves up.

Many of us do not experience victory in our lives because we have been content to live with a spiritual trickle when abundance is available. The world in which we live can drain us dry. Since we interact with carnally-minded people daily, it is easy to be influenced by this mindset. Worship gives us a respite from the world. It reminds us that we have been set apart even as we must navigate the world's dangers. During our worship time, we focus on God and matters of the spirit, which brings us life and peace.

You can practice worship in the following ways: through corporate (formal) worship, through relationships, and through your pursuit of the purpose to which God has called you.

Corporate worship is the one with which most of us are familiar: church attendance. Approach your worship services in a new way—with expectation. Observe each aspect of the service as though viewing it through the eyes of a child; focusing on God, not on how others perceive you.

Listen to the voice of the Holy Spirit as He instructs you on how to please God; if He says *sing*, then sing. If He says *dance*, then dance. If you approach worship in this way, one thing that you can count on is that church will never be boring. You will be engaged, alive, and connected to God.

The next means to practice worship is through the relationships in your life. We tend to have too many relationships that are just superficial. But God is calling us to form deep, authentic relationships with others so that He can demonstrate His love to them through us. He wants us to be "Jesus with skin on," reaching out to others to meet genuine needs, just as he did. If we take the time to receive His love through worship, then we will be able to give to others out of the overflow.

The final type of worship I will discuss is worshiping God through your life's purpose. One of my favorite quotes reads: "Our life is a gift from God; what we do with it is our gift back to Him." Are you fully using the talents He has given you and are you engaged in the purpose to which He has called you? If not, then you need to seek God's will for your life and strive to fulfill it.

Even if you can't make a grand gesture, like dropping everything and caring for the poor in Calcutta like Mother Theresa, you can give food to a homeless person if God has called you to minister to the poor. Your goal is to do the best you can with the resources God has given you.

God blesses you with gifts and talents so that you can be a blessing to others. When you are out in the world and making a difference for God, then you experience abundance. When you don't, you experience poverty of the spirit, which can create the ideal conditions for destructive attitudes and behaviors to take up residence inside you.

To end our review of worship, consider the types of worship mentioned. Is one type of worship lacking in your life? Are all of them? Your goal should be to include at least one type of worship in your life daily. We serve an awesome, gracious God. We need to take time regularly to declare both publicly and privately: "He is worthy."

WORD

As believers, we cannot live a life of effectiveness for God without knowing what His word says about the problems we confront. Diligent study of the bible adds life to every spiritual strategy we have studied: our prayer, our praise, and our worship.

When I first accepted Christ, I thought that I could continue to live the way I had been living before salvation. Nothing could be further from the truth! I have since discovered that there is a whole dimension to Christian living that few ever talk about. I learned that you can experience joy and contentment in even the most difficult times; I found out that you don't have to be a slave to your appetites because you can triumph over them through Christ.

So how can you attain these benefits? You can start by owning a bible translation that is easy for you to understand and study it regularly. Although I owned a King James Version of the bible for years, I didn't study it because I couldn't get past the Old English pronouns. I found the *New* King James Version, which I now use for most of my studies. This version has replaced the "thee" and "thous" with "you" and "yours." I recommend this version for study, but you may still need a copy of the original King James Version since many churches continue to use that version for worship services.

To get you started with your study, here are some scriptures that are relevant to making your health vision a reality. Each of these scriptures are taken from the New King James version of the bible. Meditate on them regularly and allow them to renew your mind:

3 John 1:2

"Beloved, I pray that in all respects you may prosper and be in good health, just as your soul prospers."

Romans 14:17

"...for the kingdom of God is not eating and drinking, but righteousness and peace and joy in the Holy Spirit."

Psalm 107:9

"For He has satisfied the thirsty soul, and the hungry soul He has filled with what is good."

Hebrews 12:11

"All discipline for the moment seems not to be joyful, but sorrowful; yet to those who have been trained by it, afterwards it yields the peaceful fruit of righteousness."

Galatians 5: 1

"It was for freedom that Christ set us free; So keep standing firm and do not be subject again to a yoke of slavery."

Isaiah 40:31

"Those who wait for the LORD will gain new strength; they will mount up with wings like eagles, they will run and not get tired, they will walk and not become weary."

2 Corinthians 5:17

"Therefore if anyone is in Christ, he is a new creature; the old things passed away; behold, new things have come."

Philipians 1:6

"For I am confident of this very thing, that He who began a good work in you will perfect it until the day of Christ Jesus."

With regular practice of P^2W^2 God will cultivate spiritual fruit within you, which is love, joy, peace, patience, kindness, goodness, faithfulness, gentleness, and self-control (Galatians 5:22-23). It's yours for the taking as long as you allow God's spirit to reign in your life. You don't have to go it alone. Connect with your Creator as your source several times a day and see how much difference is made in how you handle all of life's challenges— including those pertaining to your weight and health.

Small Steps Action Plan - Knowing Your True Source

Place a checkmark next to the actions you are willing to take to strengthen yourself spiritually.

Review this list once a week to be sure you are following through on your decision.

❑ Start my day with a minimum of 15 minutes of prayer.

❑ Readily forgive those who have hurt me, knowingly or unknowingly.

❑ Write down seven things each day for which to praise God for 31 days.

❑ Practice worship through church attendance, building solid relationships with others, and by walking in my God-given purpose.

❑ Initiate a regimen of regular bible study.

Chapter 3: Renewing the Mind

"The man who acquires the ability to take full possession of his own mind may take possession of anything else to which he is justly entitled."

–Andrew Carnegie, Industrialist

Have you ever heard the saying, "If you do what you've always done, you'll always get what you've always got?" Thinking the same thoughts will yield the same actions. If you want to improve your health and lose weight, you need to open your mind to new ways of thinking and acting. As speaker and author Joyce Meyer so eloquently teaches, "Where the mind goes, the man follows." That goes for the woman, too!

In many ways, your brain is like a computer; it has many programs "installed" that help you perform certain tasks. For example, you have a 'brushing my teeth' program and a 'styling my hair' program. When you were a child you had to concentrate to do these things properly but as an adult, you have done them so many times that doing them properly has become automatic.

Whether you know it or not, you also have a mental program that is keeping you overweight. You can't have habits that are controlling your life without having thoughts that support them. In this chapter we will review what you need to do to alter these thoughts so that they will support your efforts rather than sabotage them.

YOUR BRAIN: ALLY OR ENEMY?

When you are working to change your thoughts and habits, know that God designed two parts of your brain to come into play:

- The Limbic system, which is the seat of your emotions and is responsible for attention and memories

- The Neocortex, which is responsible for reasoning and judgment

If you made a fist with your left hand and placed your right hand on top of it, then your Limbic system would be housed in the fist and your Neocortex would be the hand on top.

When trying to change habits, many of us only focus on logic, giving ourselves statistics and logical reasons as to why we should change. Those activities speak to the Neocortex part of your brain. However, if you do not additionally speak to the Limbic system part of your brain, you will likely fail. Why? The Limbic system is responsible for protecting you. Have you ever heard of 'fight or flight?' This is the body's response to perceived danger and helps determine whether you should fight the source of danger or run from it.

One way the Limbic system determines whether an activity is dangerous is to inquire:

- Is the activity familiar to me?

  - If the answer is yes, the activity is usually seen as safe.
  - If the answer is no, the activity is seen as a potential source of pain and your Limbic system will help you resist doing it.

This is important because the easiest way for the Limbic system to perform its job in keeping you safe is to *maintain the habits you already have.*

Let's say that you've decided to start an exercise program by running. The first morning, you wake up at 5 o'clock in the morning, put on your jogging sneakers and charge out of the house. No warm-up for you; instead you decide to run full blast. You convince yourself that you are getting healthy and energetic by doing this. This keeps you motivated—for a while.

After about two weeks, you are lying in bed at 5 o'clock in the morning. The bed feels so good and warm. You imagine going out into the cold morning air. You imagine how uncomfortable that would feel. You think about the shin splints that you've started to develop and how painful they are. You turn over in bed. Maybe you will just sleep in this one time and start back tomorrow.

Of course, you don't start back tomorrow. In fact, before you know it, you've completely abandoned your program. What went wrong? Your Limbic system convinced you to stop your exercise program by associating pleasure to staying in bed, and pain to going out jogging.

So even if your inactivity habits aren't serving you, your Limbic system thinks they are good because it has associated pleasure to them. Plus you have engaged in them for so long that it sees these habits as safe.

Now you might be thinking "How do I change my brain so that it supports my health goal?" You can do this by speaking the Limbic system's language. This part of your brain responds to three primary factors: consistency, passion, and rewards. Just think of the acronym CPR. Let's discuss the 'C' first.

Consistency is important because your brain loves habit patterns. When you practice a habit over and over, pathways are created in the brain. Once a pathway is built, all you do is start your usual activity and your brain drives you the rest of the way. God is such an awesome creator!

Have you ever had the experience of starting to drive to work, arriving at the appointed time, but not remembering how you got there? That is because you have taken that route so many times that you now have a pathway built in your brain that knows how to get to your job without you even having to "think" about it. This is to your advantage ...provided the pathways are leading you in the right direction.

So the key to building beneficial pathways in your mind is to practice healthy habits until they feel normal. Once they do, you know the mental pathway has been laid out. If you stop practicing the habit anytime before it starts to feel normal, you will stop the pathway construction. The key lesson here is to be consistent. Some research suggests that it takes a minimum of 30 days of consistent practice to form new habits.

Let's return to our previous 'running' example. Suppose you hadn't quit running during the second week, in spite of your brain's protest that it was too cold and too early. Somewhere around the fourth week, you notice that your brain isn't protesting as much. By week six, it isn't protesting at all. In fact, it is even starting to prompt you that you need to go ahead and get out of bed so that you can get your run in. Your Limbic system has now become your biggest ally in keeping your new habit going.

The next factor that the Limbic system loves is passion, the 'P' in our CPR acronym. Because this part of your brain is the seat of your emotions, you'll need to make sure to stay motivated when going for your weight loss goals. If you have a 'take it or leave it' attitude towards your goal, then your Limbic system will also see it as less important. Since this area of the brain is also responsible for memory, it won't waste effort trying to remember things that you've deemed unimportant. For an example, just think about any New Year's resolutions you've made in the past. How many of those were forgotten or abandoned by February 1?

One way to stay passionate about your goals is to focus on the outcome you want to achieve. In Chapter 1, I recommended that you visualize yourself as having already reached your goal twice a day. By doing this, you are convincing your Limbic system that this goal is important to you and you need its help to accomplish it.

If you don't stress your goal's importance, 'out of sight, out of mind' will be all too true for you.

The last way to speak the Limbic system's language is to use 'Rewards' (the 'R' in CPR). The Limbic system loves pleasure. Your current habits may be hard to change because not only does your brain have well-established pathways surrounding them but it also finds them pleasurable. Any experience it finds pleasurable is one it will drive you to repeat. This aspect of the Limbic system is clear evidence that God wants you to enjoy life!

However to use this knowledge to your benefit, you must make your new habits more fun than your old ones. That's why it will be critical for you to think of this process not as merely losing weight but as building health and adding joy to your life. The weight loss is just a very positive side effect.

You can make the process more pleasurable by finding your personal health "sweet spot"...willing to experiment with healthier foods, keeping the ones that taste good to you and discarding the ones that don't. If you disliked a particularly healthy food when you were a child don't assume that you still dislike it as an adult. Be willing to try it again. If you like it now then you've added some variety to your diet. If you don't you haven't lost anything.

On the physical activity side find activities that you think you might enjoy or at least would not dread. Adopt the attitude of a child; fidget, pace, skip, dance, spin...just increase your activity level in general outside of formal exercise periods. Start to think of yourself as an active, involved person.

One great reward to give yourself and increase your pleasure in your new habits at the same time is through the use of hugs. Having often watched Olympic competitions, I noticed that the coaches regularly hugged the female competitors after their routines. To reinforce positive behaviors, pick a physical means to show appreciation to yourself for a job well done. Hug yourself after every glass of water, fruit or vegetable eaten, or exercise session. If you feel self-conscious about that, then a literal pat on the back should work too.

Hugging is the best choice because studies have shown that this gesture produces a hormone called 'endorphins' in the body. This chemical makes us feel good and also increases calmness and contentment.

Other natural ways we can get our bodies to produce endorphins are through challenging but comfortable exercise sessions, and through laughter, uplifting music, delightful smells, and pleasant touch. Why not make use of these activities to make your health experience as pleasurable as possible? The greater pleasure you receive, the more the Limbic system will be your powerful ally.

YOUR ATTITUDE: HELPFUL OR HIINDRANCE?

You've probably heard the old saying that "attitude is everything." While I don't believe attitude is *everything*, it is important when it comes to losing weight. Without the right attitude, failure is guaranteed.

Here are the top four attitude-related issues that can destroy your chances of losing weight successfully—and then some ways to overcome them.

Playing "When I lose weight then I'll…" games

I formerly taught an online stress management class and 'body image' often surfaced in our discussions about self-esteem. One of my students wrote a comment that saddened me. Theresa mentioned that she was considerably overweight, but explained in great detail all the things she aspired to when she finally lost the weight.

The funny thing was that the goals she mentioned weren't outrageous ones like climbing Mount Everest; her goals were simple things like getting her hair cut in a flattering style, buying clothes that fit, and finding a job that she liked.

I was sad because she felt that she wasn't worthy of those things until the numbers on a scale said 125. Do you play those games too? If so, what is your number?

I can sympathize because I once did the same thing to myself. Instead of giving myself the unconditional love that I craved and that God has for me, I would use these games as a form of emotional blackmail. I thought that if I withheld nice things from myself, I would be motivated to do something about my weight.

It never worked. Such mind games only made me feel even worse than I had before.

Playing "if I lose weight, then I'll…" games is a form of conditional love. You wouldn't dream of telling your family and friends that you won't love them if they don't take a certain action, but you actually do that to *yourself* when you play these games.

These destructive thought patterns are also a way of putting your life on hold. Realize that you can only live life today because tomorrow isn't promised to any of us. You deserve to have God's best for your life and taking good care of yourself *now* is the ultimate way to ensure that He will bless you with good health.

Eating to cope with unpleasant emotions

How many times have you eaten something when your body wasn't hungry? If you tend to eat for emotional reasons, then the answer to that question might be, "Quite a bit." However, this must change since eating food when your body is not hungry will only cause your body to store the excess as fat.

Before you eat anything, always ask "Is my body hungry?" If the answer is 'no' then ask "Why then do I want to eat?" Your answer will reveal to you the actual need. Chances are you are feeling an unpleasant emotion that you are attempting to avoid. It takes courage to confront these emotions, but it will be necessary in achieving your goals.

The following are a few suggestions for dealing with negative emotions that have worked for myself and others:

Emotion	Suggested Ways to Cope
• Anger	• Pray, asking for God's peace and comfort to descend upon you • Pound a pillow • Go off alone and have a good scream or cry • Practice deep breathing to calm yourself down • After calming yourself, discuss the situation with the person with whom you are angry in a direct, but gentle manner. • Describe the situation that is making you angry on paper; when you are finished, crumple up the paper and flush or trash it.
• Boredom	• Take a nature walk • Visit a friend • Organize a cluttered area at home or work • Rearrange/redecorate a room in your home to better suit you • Go "people watching" or "prayer walking" at a mall or playground

• Depression (mild)	• Pray, asking for God's peace and joy to fill your spirit • Talk to a friend or counselor • Listen to spiritually uplifting music or sing praise songs • Take a walk in the sunshine and fresh air • Start a praise journal and count your blessings • Perform an act of random kindness for someone else
• Frustration	• Play with a child's toy such as a yoyo, paddleball, or bouncing ball • Put on one of your favorite CDs and dance around • Write down what is bothering you and put it aside; go for a walk and talk it over with God. Read the paper again when you come back. You are bound to see things from a new perspective
• Loneliness	• Talk to God...out loud • Visit/call a friend • Volunteer to visit the sick or a shut-in
• Procrastination	• Create a goals list - what do you want to do with your life? • Do the simplest thing on the list **now** • Do the thing on the list that

	will make you feel best for having completed it • Try to discover the reasons behind your procrastination. Usually these reasons are either a fear of failure or even success
• Tiredness	• Take a nap or turn in early in the evening • Soak your feet in warm water and use a foot scrub to wash them (peppermint foot scrub is great) • Use reviving scents in your environment, such as orange and lemon • Practice breathing/relaxation exercises to unwind

Procrastinating on important tasks

In talking with many people who have weight problems, I have discovered that, more often than not, their weight is not the only area that has spun out of control. They are also usually living with financial challenges, relationship trauma, or a disorganized living environment. All of these issues can signal a life out of balance.

I mentioned earlier that I had significant debt when my weight was at its height. For a long time I ignored my debt because it was a painful issue. I would put bills in a box, unopened. I let the answering machine handle all of my calls because I didn't want to talk to the creditors about my late payments.

I had dysfunctional romantic relationships, and my house stayed cluttered and messy. I didn't have enough energy to do even the most basic life tasks. Can you relate?

I have a quick exercise for you: Stop reading for a moment and take a look at the state of your house. Is your home free of clutter? Are your bills in order? Individually, these seem like small things, but failure to take care of them collectively points to a reason why you might be having a hard time shedding pounds.

Losing weight requires discipline, planning, and organization. These are the same skills that are required to keep your house in order and to manage your financial life.

In my case, I discovered that I would often eat as a form of procrastination. What do you need to do that you have been avoiding, besides your weight? You might begin tackling that area to give you confidence to then take on your health issues.

For example, if your house is cluttered and unkempt, begin by deciding to clean up a small corner. Just grab a grocery bag and start throwing away things that you no longer need. Better yet, if you have items in good shape that you don't use, then put those aside for donation to a charity organization such as *Goodwill* or the *Salvation Army*. Not only will you help someone else by taking on this task but you will also increase your confidence and diligence. Once you improve one area, chances are you will address others and gain a better quality of life overall.

Problems delaying gratification

Delaying gratification is simply the ability to say 'no' to a pleasurable activity now in favor of greater enjoyment and reward in the future. It doesn't mean saying no forever but simply "no for now."

For example, let's say that you love eating brownies but know that you have a hard time controlling yourself around them. You go to a buffet and there they are: lovely brownies. One way to practice your ability to delay gratification is to simply say to yourself "I'm not going to have those right now. I'll eat my dinner and if

I'm still hungry I may eat one later." Very likely, by the time "later" arrives, you won't want the brownie anymore.

You can also try delaying by the clock. This method is a good one to try if you find yourself often eating second helpings at meals. After you've eaten your first helping and are about to reload, tell yourself "I'll wait for 10 minutes before having more. If I still want one I will get it." Like in the first example, the delay is usually all you will need to ensure that you don't end up eating more food than your body needs simply because of habit.

So in order to succeed with your weight loss goals, you should turn the four hindrance attitudes into ones that help you:

- You take care of yourself *now*

- You take care of important tasks *now*

- You face unpleasant emotions in a constructive manner *now*

- You eat foods that are less healthy or problematic for you *later*

With these attitude shifts, you will find that your weight loss efforts will be more enjoyable and effective.

Small Steps Action Plan - Renewing the Mind

Place a checkmark next to the actions you are willing to take for renewing your mind to support your efforts.

Review this list once a week to be sure you are following through on your decision.

❑ I've decided to be consistent with my new health habits.

❑ I continually motivate myself by staying passionate about mastering my goals.

❑ I reward myself not only for achieving my weight/size goals but for each positive health habit I practice (hugs, pats on the back).

❑ I practice delayed gratification techniques regarding eating habits that don't align with my weight loss goals.

❑ I do nice things for myself *now* instead of waiting until I lose weight.

❑ I take action *now* on important tasks instead of putting things off, even if I just take one small step forward each day towards accomplishing them.

❑ I face unpleasant emotions and practice constructive ways to deal with them rather than bury them under food.

Part 2

Building a Better Body

Chapter 4: Eating Well on a Budget

"Eating is not merely a material pleasure. Eating well gives a spectacular joy to life and contributes immensely to goodwill and happy companionship. It is of great importance to the morale."

– Elsa Schiaparelli, Italian Designer

Enjoying your food is essential for attaining your ideal weight. In the previous chapter, you learned that building pleasure into the process will help you enlist the Limbic system to keeping your new health habits for life.

If you are a veteran dieter, just think about the times you *made* yourself eat food that you didn't like just because it promised quick weight loss. You probably didn't stick with the regimen for very long. Fortunately there are many foods that taste good but will also help you stay with your weight loss goals.

Think of good health as a wall of defense around your body. Without that wall of defense, disease is free to enter and wreck havoc with your life. In this chapter we will discuss how you can have the best of all worlds: lose weight, get healthy, avoid disease, look better, feel great, and save money. First, we will review how much unhealthy habits are actually costing you.

THE HIGH COST OF POOR EATING HABITS

We know now that many diseases are lifestyle related and arise from poor eating habits and inactivity. For example, obesity has a serious monetary cost; According to the Center of Disease Control (CDC), losing just 10% of excess body weight can reduce your medical costs by $2,000 to $5,300 over your lifetime. That means that if you weigh 180, losing just 18 pounds can ultimately make a great difference in your finances.

Here are some other savings you could realize from adopting healthier habits and achieving your ideal weight:

- You could save over $1,000 in a year if you eliminate $3 of daily spending on junk or fast food.

- You could spend less on clothing since plus-sized clothing costs 10-15% more than regular-sized clothing.

- You could ultimately save on health services and medications costs; according to a study by the Rand Corporation, obese people spend 36% more on health services and 77% more on medications than people who have maintained their optimal weight.

You can also save up to $468 per year by eating only enough to feed the body's needs. Let's explore that concept in more detail.

MINDFUL EATING

One way to ensure that you are eating only to satisfy your body's need is to practice a concept called SANE eating.

The acronym S.A.N.E stands for:

- Start when you are hungry
- Appreciate every bite
- No food is forbidden
- End when signaled

Start When You Are Hungry

You may not have allowed yourself to become physically hungry in a while, but eating to satisfy bodily hunger is the way God designed us in the first place.

Going forward, *pause* whenever you have the desire to eat. Check your stomach and ask, "Is my body hungry?" If the answer is "maybe" or "no" then you should not eat yet.

Do the following instead:

- For "maybe" answers, drink a glass of water, brush your teeth, or chew on a stick of sugarless gum. Make sure the gum has an intense flavor, such as mint or peppermint. Wait 10 minutes and then check again.

  Do not merely sit during those 10 minutes; find another task to occupy your time. Preferably, the task should be a physical one, such as going for a walk, tidying up, or engaging in a hobby. The goal is to distract your mind (where the tempting thoughts are coming from) and get focused on your body.

  After the 10 minutes is over, ask yourself the question again, "Is my body hungry?" By then, you should have either a definite "yes" or "no" answer.

- For "no" answers, ask yourself another question, "Why then do I want to eat?" Use the suggested methods for coping with emotional eating that were outlined in the previous chapter.

Another way to tell if your body is hungry is to place your hands on your stomach and rate your hunger according to the following scale:

5 – I have no hunger pangs at all; in fact, I am full from a previous meal.

4 – I have no hunger pangs at all; I'm not full, but I am satisfied with the moderate amount of food in my stomach.

3 – My stomach feels vaguely uneasy. I have a little food in my stomach, and I could eat something.

2 – I feel hunger pangs; I have no food in my stomach. I definitely need to eat.

1 – I feel strong hunger pangs; I have a headache and I feel slightly nauseous. I can't think straight; I want to eat everything in sight.

Your goal is balance —not to experience the severe hunger of level 1 and not to eat when you are at levels 4 and 5. If you allow yourself to get as low as a level 1, then your brain will not care what type of food you get as long as you eat. It thinks you are starving and will likely crave high fat, high sugar foods to raise your blood sugar level up as quickly as possible.

On the other hand, if you eat at levels 4 and 5, you will be giving your body food that it doesn't need. Since it's not needed, this food will likely be stored in your fat cells.

Ideally, you want to eat when your hunger level is either 2 or 3. At that level, your body does require food, plus you will have the presence of mind to make wise decisions as to what to eat.

Appreciate every bite

Have you ever wolfed food down so fast that you didn't even recall eating? Taking time to sit down and savor a meal may seem like an indulgence, but it is an important component to your weight loss efforts. Here is why.

An area in our brain called the *appestat* monitors our food intake and sends signals to indicate when we have had enough to eat. But the appestat is a bit of a slowpoke; it takes 20 minutes of eating before registering satisfaction. Many of us hurriedly consume our meals within the space of 5-10 minutes. If your brain has not signaled that you have had enough, then it is quite possible for you to eat *twice* as much as your body really needs.

So, you want to take time to enjoy your meals, silently thanking God for each bite, and giving the appestat time to do its job. One other benefit with slowing down is that your digestion will improve. Food digestion really begins in the mouth. To digest properly, your food should be in nearly a liquid state before you swallow it. Your teeth were made to grind the food into manageable pieces with the saliva aiding the process. If you don't take time to really chew your food, then you are setting yourself up for indigestion and acid reflux.

Finally, you want to relax and make your mealtimes as stress free as possible. If you are stressed, your body manufactures *cortisol,* as mentioned in an earlier chapter. Among other functions, cortisol contributes to the storage of fat around your midsection. By taking time to savor your meals, you can help relieve stress and prevent this mechanism from taking hold. In addition, you will get more pleasure out of your meals, so you will be satisfied with eating less.

No foods are forbidden

If you are accustomed to restrictive eating you might be surprised by this guideline. You can have *any* food you want.

Having said this, a smart strategy would be to become educated on the effects that certain foods have on your body. Some foods have a positive effect and will lean your body down and some foods will have a destructive one and make it more likely that you will store fat.

Since your body constantly remakes itself based on your food intake, the beverages you drink, and the movements you make, you want to consider your choices carefully. If you want to build a high quality body, you must give it high quality building materials.

While you won't "forbid" yourself to have certain foods, realize that some foods will slow down your weight loss goal and make it harder for you to make healthy choices. These foods are:

- Sugars
- White flour products
- White rice

These foods are simple carbohydrates, which mean that the body can break them down quickly into glucose (also known as sugar). When your body breaks down these foods, it releases the sugar into your bloodstream. The body produces insulin, a hormone that is designed to bring your blood sugar down by moving the sugar into your muscle cells where it can be burned as fuel.

In some cases, the blood sugar is lowered rapidly. This causes a domino effect:

1. With a lowered blood sugar, your body wants to bring you back into balance as quickly as possible. Food cravings are triggered.

2. You crave foods that are high in fat and sugar. Your body sees this as a necessary measure, thinking it is in a crisis state and these foods will bring your blood sugar up quickly.

3. The insulin that was produced by your body also encourages the storage of fat, so the extra food you consumed will likely be stored as "extra padding."

In addition to fostering weight gain, these types of foods make it more difficult to make wise choices. Your thinking becomes unfocused and you experience mood swings when your blood sugar fluctuates to extremes.

This makes it more likely that you will make poor food selections.

A wise practice to adopt is paying attention to how you feel after you eat certain foods. Did your body like the food that you ate or not? Some clues that your body may not like a particular food are:

- You feel drugged, numb, or suffer from "brain fog"
- You feel bloated or nauseous
- You feel sluggish or sleepy

The food you eat should *give* you energy, not deplete it. If a food affects you in a negative way, start recording the reaction. This will give you a helpful guide so that you can start eating food that your whole body likes, not just your tongue. It will also assist you in deciding to limit foods that affect your body negatively. The best strategy would be to eat them only on rare occasions or to practice portion control when you do eat them.

End when signaled

When your body has had enough to eat, you experience a nice, pleasant feeling. You don't have hunger pangs and you feel comfortable, but not full. On the hunger scale, you are at a level 4. This "signal point" can also be called the *fat point* because if you eat more than your body needs, what happens? Exceeding your body's calorie needs for the day will cause the body to store the excess as fat, as mentioned earlier.

To ensure that you stop eating when signaled, you will need to pay attention while you are eating. That means when you are eating, you should only be *eating*, not multi-tasking with T.V. watching or reading a book.

Eat until the point when your body is *no longer hungry*. Three to four bites after that is usually the signal point for most people, but you will need to monitor yourself to discover your own point. When you reach it, stop eating. If you continue, you will enter the fat-storing zone.

Take the attitude that you would rather store the extra food in a container and freeze it for later than store it on your body. Eating appropriate amounts is the first strategy to lose weight and save money.

FOODS TO EAT TO LOSE WEIGHT

The next strategy to trim down and save bucks is to primarily eat those foods that establish health in the body and practice wise shopping strategies to purchase these foods.

Those foods are:

- Fruits and vegetables (bright colors are best since they contain more flavanoids, compounds known to play a role in the prevention of heart disease and certain cancers)

- Whole grains/starchy vegetables (pasta, bread, rice, cereal, sweet potatoes, corn)

- Protein (lean meat, fish, beans, and low fat dairy or soy-based products)

The following chart explains why these foods support your weight loss efforts (some of the content that follows was adapted from the *MoneyWise Weight Loss Practical Guide*):

Food category	Why important in weight loss
Fruits and Vegetables	Supply the body with an abundance of 'B' vitamins, which aid thyroid function and help the body convert food to energy. • Good sources of B vitamins include leafy green vegetables, cabbage, bananas, cauliflower, cucumber, oranges, tangerines, grapefruit, and lemons.

	Certain fruits and vegetables also supply 'C' vitamins, which help the body convert glucose (sugar) to energy in the cells. • Good sources of C vitamins include broccoli, green peppers, kiwi fruit, strawberries, oranges, and cabbage. Fruits and vegetables also contain fiber, a non-digestible component of plant foods. Fiber makes you feel full on fewer calories. • Good sources of fiber includes dark green leafy vegetables, tomatoes, peas, carrots, apples, and pears.
Whole grains/starchy vegetables	Great source of fiber and other nutrients. It also aids digestion and helps prevent constipation. Research also shows that eating complex carbohydrates makes you feel more calm and relaxed. Examples include: • Sweet potatoes, corn, whole grain bread, brown or wild rice, whole grain pastas, cooked cereals
Protein	Helps support muscle growth and repair. Muscles burn more calories at rest than does fat. In addition, eating lean protein

	can reduce your appetite, which can reduce your caloric intake overall, plus it makes you feel more mentally alert. Examples include: • Beans, fish, chicken, turkey, meat substitutes (tofu-based) low-fat dairy products
Water	You may be eating when you are really thirsty since the same part of the brain controls both hunger and thirst. Taking in enough water ensures that you aren't consuming calories without cause. According to research, it can also prevent headaches and increase your energy since dehydration is one cause of lethargy.

The following is the recommended number of servings from each food group each day to attain your ideal weight:

Food/beverage	Daily serving recommendations
Fruits and vegetables	Minimum 5 servings of vegetables Minimum 2 servings of fruit
Whole grains/starchy vegetables	Maximum 3 servings per day

Protein	3-4 servings per day
Water/fluids	Minimum 8 glasses

Note: The recommended servings above are guidelines for women; the recommended servings for men are as follows:

- Six servings of vegetables per day

- Three servings of fruit per day

- Four servings of whole grain/starch per day

- Four to five servings of protein per day

As an example, here is how women can obtain the recommended servings in a typical day's menu, fruits and vegetables in particular. With this pattern, you will eat approximately five times a day, which is a real bonus if you enjoy eating! Eating frequent, small meals is also the pattern that most medical professionals recommend to keep your blood sugar stable:

Breakfast
- 1 cup 1% milk
- 1 cup oatmeal
- 1/2 banana

Lunch
- 3 oz. oven fried fish
- 1/2 c. sweet potato fries
- 2 cups of light coleslaw

Dinner
- 3 oz roast chicken
- 1 small corn on the cob
- 1 c. steamed green beans

Morning Snack
- 1 cup carrot and celery strips

Afternoon snack
- 1/2 banana
- A miniature chocolate bar*

*Tip: If you crave chocolate, try some of the low sugar/low carbohydrate varieties on the market periodically. Read the label and limit the amount you eat to one serving. However, if you find yourself consistently eating more than that, then this is likely a problem food for you and you should save it for special occasions.

PRACTICAL PORTION SIZES

Now let's describe an appropriate portion size for each of the food groups. Whenever possible, I will describe the size in a way that is easy to see. A typical vegetable/fruit serving size fits in the palm of your hand:

- 1 cup of raw vegetables
- ½ cup of cooked vegetables (½ cup is also about the size of ½ orange):
- ¾ cup of vegetable juice
- 1 medium whole fruit (apple, orange, pear)
- ½ large fruit (like a grapefruit)
- ½ c of canned, chopped, or cooked fruit
- ½ cup fruit juice
- ¼ of dried fruit

When it comes to fruit servings, always strive to select the actual fruit rather than juices or dried fruit. The water and fiber content will fill you up so that you are satisfied without caloric excesses. Since eating more fruits and vegetables will be your secret weapon in shedding pounds, you will receive more ideas on practical ways to increase your servings of these foods in upcoming pages.

A typical serving of whole grains/starchy vegetables includes:

- ½ cup of wild or brown rice
- ½ of a whole wheat bagel or bun
- ½ cup of whole grain pasta
- ½ cup of cooked cereal (for example, oatmeal or cream of wheat)
- 1 slice of whole grain bread
- 1 small corn on the cob
- 1 small sweet potato

Unlike the simple carbohydrates I mentioned earlier (white flour products, white rice, etc) these carbohydrates are more complex. The fiber they contain slows the rate at which food is broken down into glucose, which means that you won't experience severe blood sugar fluctuations.

The following are suggested protein serving sizes:

- 3 oz. lean meat, fish, or poultry (about the size of your palm; fingers don't count)
- 1 egg or 1/2 c. egg substitute

- 1 cup of low fat milk (1% milk)
- 1 piece of part-skim mozzarella string cheese
- 1 ½ oz. of other low fat cheese (cheddar, American, Swiss); this is about the size of your index finger
- 1 cup of low fat yogurt (or small container)
- ½ c. cooked beans
- 1 TBSP peanut butter

Your water servings could be obtained as follows:

- 2 cups of water before breakfast

- 2 cups of water before lunch

- 2 cups of water before dinner

- 2 cups of water before bedtime (drink at least 2 hours before bedtime, otherwise you might have to get up during the night with unexpected bathroom trips).

Other fluids can also count toward your water intake, such as low-fat milk and juices. The most important thing is to be sure that you are drinking adequate amounts daily.

An easy way to control your portions when preparing your plate is to use the following concept as recommended in the Idaho Plate Method:

1. Divide half of your dinner plate and fill it with vegetables.

2. Split the other half in two. One half of this portion is for whole grains/starchy vegetables.

3. The other half is for lean protein.

So your plate should look like this:

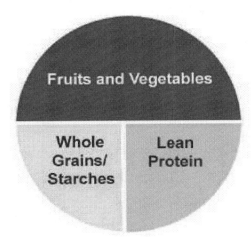

WISE SHOPPING STRATEGIES FOR FOOD

To save money on food, it's recommended that you start with the following guidelines:

- Figure how much money you will spend **before** going to the store.
- Shop with a list. Shopping lists help you shorten your time in the store; statistics show that the longer time you spend in the grocery store, the more you tend to spend.
- Always shop with a calculator to help you stay within your budget. Check prices carefully at the cash register to avoid being overcharged when items occasionally ring up with the wrong prices.

- Focus on foods located on or near the walls (store perimeter). This is usually where the healthier foods are. Processed foods high in fat, salt, starch, and sugar are usually located in the center aisles, so shop these aisles last and don't stay in them very long!

- Never shop when you are hungry; everything looks good, plus you will end up buying items that you do not need.

You might create a shopping list as follows:

1. Scour your cabinets and refrigerator to see what food you have available.
2. Check any grocery store sales and circulars for nutritious foods that are good buys. Add those to your list.
3. Decide what meals you're going to prepare based on the food you already have and healthy items on sale.

   Think about the main course first and then plan side items around it. Try to plan meals around meat alternatives at least twice a week such as eggs, soy-based meat substitutes, dried beans, or peas. Meat is usually the most expensive food item you purchase, so using less of it will automatically save you money.

   Add any missing ingredients for a meal to your list.

4. Select what additional food you need for breakfast, lunches and snacks. Complete your list.

Saving on Fruit and Vegetables

The following fruits and vegetables are usually good buys since they are available all year long:

- Apples
- Bananas
- Carrots
- Cabbage
- Celery

- Greens
- Lettuce (Iceberg)
- Onions
- Oranges
- Sweet potatoes

Bagged, cut up greens (turnips, collards, mustards, etc) are more expensive; save money by purchasing bunched greens and chop them yourself. The same rules apply for fruits; you will pay more if they are pre cut.

Buy other fresh fruits/vegetables in season. "In season" means that the item is plentiful and at the peak of freshness. In general, here is a list of fruits and vegetables and the seasons in which they tend to cost less due to wider availability:

Season	Fruit/Vegetable	
Spring	Apricots	New Potatoes
	Artichoke	Pineapple
	Asparagus	Rhubarb
	Avocado	Spinach
	Carrots	Spring Baby Lettuce Mixes
	Collards	

	Mango	Strawberries
	Mustard Greens	Sugar Snap and Snow Peas
		Vidalia Onions
Summer	Beets	Nectarines
	Blackberries	Peaches
	Blueberries	Plums
	Broccoli	Raspberries
	Corn	Summer Squash
	Cucumber	Tomatoes
	Eggplant	Watermelon
	Green Beans	Zucchini
Fall	Acorn Squash	Parsnips
	Apples	Pears
	Butternut Squash	Pomegranate
	Cauliflower	Pumpkin
	Garlic	Sweet Potatoes
	Grapes	Swiss Chard
	Mushrooms	
Winter	Chestnuts	Oranges and Tangerines
	Grapefruit	Radishes
	Kale	Rutabagas
	Lemons	Turnips

When shopping, stock up on fruit and vegetables that tend to last a week or longer, such as apples, oranges, pears, melons, nectarines, cabbage, turnips, broccoli, cauliflower, and onions.

Store most fresh vegetables in the refrigerator; greens should be stored in the refrigerator in a plastic bag. Placing a paper towel in with them will absorb moisture and can help them last longer (replace the towel with a dry one when it becomes damp). Store bananas, garlic, onions, potatoes, and tomatoes at room temperature.

If you have access to a Farmers Market or roadside stand, you can purchase fruits and vegetables there to save additional money.

Frozen vegetables are your next best buy if you can't buy fresh. Large bags are usually cheaper overall than small ones. Also, vegetables without sauces are cheaper than vegetables with sauces.

Good frozen vegetable buys usually are:

- Broccoli
- Corn
- Mixed vegetables
- Peas
- Peas and carrots
- Spinach
- Turnip greens

Canned vegetables should be your last choice due to high salt content and vitamin depletion. If you buy them, purchase the low sodium versions or rinse them thoroughly before using.

Be sure to buy canned fruit either packed in water or in its own juice, not packed in syrup (even "light" syrup).

Purchase a mix of fresh, frozen, and canned vegetables. Always use the fresh fruits/vegetables first, making a habit of checking your vegetable bin every day.

To avoid waste, keep fruits and vegetables readily available. Have a fruit bowl on the kitchen table or counter filled with fruits that your family likes, such as bananas, apples and oranges—all usually popular with children. You can also keep a vegetable plate of carrots, cucumbers, and tomato slices in the refrigerator with low fat ranch dressing for snacking.

Another tip to use more vegetables is to sneak them into the foods you cook. Use leftover ones in a stir fry or salad. Add extra vegetables to spaghetti sauce, soups, stews, and casseroles. Add fruit to yogurt or cereal. You can also add extra vegetable servings simply by buying the "chunky" versions of salsa and spaghetti sauce.

Saving on Whole Grains and Starchy Vegetables

When you purchase a bread or grain product, always read the list of ingredients and look for the word "whole." If an ingredient just says "wheat flour" then it is just white flour that has had molasses or another substance added to give it a brown color.

Here are some tips for saving money on these items:

- Check and compare the cost per unit displayed on the shelf labels for items you want to buy. For example, a box of pasta that costs 80 cents for a 10 oz box (8 cents per unit) is a better buy than one costing 72 cents for a 6 oz box (12 cents per unit).

- Items at eye level on the shelves usually cost more. Scan lower and upper shelves for cheaper whole grain items.

  Limit buying items displayed at the cash register or on the "end caps," which are special displays at the end of grocery store aisles. Since manufacturers pay grocery stores to feature their products on end caps, these are generally higher profit items.

- Buy the Sunday paper and look for coupons for healthy items. But only use them if the brand name price with the coupon is cheaper than the store brand without the discount. Store brands are usually less expensive anyway.

- Buy multi-packs of rolls and bagels rather than individual ones (from bakeries, etc).

- Day-old bread can be cheaper and frozen to extend its shelf life.

- Buy regular brown rice and oatmeal instead of the instant or flavored varieties since they cost more.

- Canned corn and sweet potatoes are usually good buys. Rinse canned vegetables thoroughly to remove excess salt.

- Finally, avoid impulse shopping by buying only what you really need. Snack chips, candy, cookies, and items like them are considered a "want" item, not a need. Save them for rare occasions to save money and your waist line.

Saving on protein

- Compare the cost per pound of whole meats versus those that are already cut up. For example, buying a whole chicken and slicing it yourself is more cost effective than buying the individual parts.

- Stock up on chicken and turkey when they are on sale; a good time to do so is around holidays like Thanksgiving and Christmas.

- Frozen Whiting or Alaskan Pollock are usually wise buys in seafood. Canned tuna or salmon are also good alternatives. Wait for sales on fresh fish.

If you buy beef, get the cheaper cuts like ground beef (but avoid pre-made hamburger patties since these are more expensive), round, or chuck. You can reduce the fat in ground beef by as much as 50% if you use the following rinsing process:

1. Brown the ground beef for 8-10 minutes until no longer pink.

2. Microwave 4 cups of water on High for 5-6 minutes.

3. Pour the excess fat off of the cooked ground beef. Transfer the ground beef with a slotted spoon to a plate lined with 3-4 white paper towels.

4. Allow it to sit for 1-2 minutes to drain the fat.

5. Blot the ground beef crumbles with more paper towels to absorb additional fat.

6. Transfer the beef only to a colander in the sink. Pour the hot water over the beef and then allow it to sit for 5 minutes to drain.

Use the beef crumbles in recipes like spaghetti, chili, soup, or stews.

You may need to marinate less tender cuts of meat like round or chuck steak with an oil-free marinate for 1-2 hours. Marinate the meat in a plastic bag in the refrigerator for easy clean up.

Do not use the marinating solution to baste the meat while cooking; you risk re-contaminating cooked meat with bacteria that may have been on the raw meat.

- Prepare soups, stews, and casseroles more often, decreasing the amount of meat and increasing the vegetables.

- Plan to have two or more meatless meals per week using beans for protein. This practice can save hundreds of dollars each year. Recall that meat is usually the most expensive item you purchase. Great meatless meals could include vegetable soup, pasta salad, or vegetarian chili, or pizza.

Small Steps Action Plan - Eating Well on a Budget

Place a checkmark next to the actions you are willing to take to eat well in order to get fit.

Review this list once a week to be sure you are following through on your decision.

❑   I will most often eat when my *body* is hungry.

❑   If I am not hungry, I will pause and ask myself why I want to eat. I then practice alternative actions instead.

❑   I plan to give myself 20 minutes to eat and thankfully enjoy my meals.

❑   I'll reassure myself that no food is forbidden to me.

❑   I will pay attention to how certain foods make me feel. If a food makes me feel bloated, drugged, or sleepy, I limit it in my diet.

❑   I eat until my body is no longer hungry, not to the point of fullness.

❑   I will ingest foods in the right portion sizes.

❑   I intend to eat the recommended number of servings for fruits/vegetables, whole grains/starchy vegetables, and lean protein.

❑   I plan to practice at least three of the recommendations for saving money on food.

Chapter 5: Healthy Meals on the Go

"If we're not willing to settle for junk living, we certainly shouldn't settle for junk food."

— Sally Edwards, Athlete and Speaker

Taking back your temple is all about quality and balance. You want to ensure that the majority of the foods you eat give you the most nutrition at the best price; at the same time, you want to enjoy your life—still allowing yourself to have the less healthy foods you love, but saving them for special occasions. It's not about living a diet; it's about living an abundant life. Eating is a necessary part of life and should be pleasurable.

One of the most efficient ways to shed pounds and get healthy is making fruits and vegetables the cornerstone of your diet. In the book of Genesis God told Adam that he could have every herb that yields seed and every tree whose fruit yields seed for food. Since He only later allowed humans to have meat, seemingly foods that come from the ground represent God's first and best. Water is also the body's preferred source of fluid.

In addition to choosing foods that will give you maximum nutrition, you want to prepare them in the healthiest ways possible. This chapter gives you some guidelines on healthy food preparation. Since you will probably also have situations in which you will need to eat away from home, we will also explore some principles for making nutritious food selections.

FAST AND HEALTHY MEALS

Preparing healthy meals starts with ensuring that you keep your cabinets and refrigerator stocked with staple foods that can serve as ingredients for many meals. Here are some non-perishable items that you should keep on hand:

In the cabinet/pantry

- Canned tomatoes
- Canned fruit (in its own juice)
- Canned beans and peas (kidney beans, black beans, black-eyed peas, lentils, etc.)
- Canned corn
- Canned, vegetable-rich soups (look for low sodium, lower fat varieties
- Jars of chunky spaghetti or marinara sauce
- Canned tuna or salmon
- Canned chicken
- Powdered non-fat milk
- Whole wheat pancake mix
- Oatmeal

- Brown rice
- Whole grain pastas (spaghetti, macaroni)
- Cornmeal mix
- Chicken, beef, or vegetable broth, bouillon cubes, or dried onion soup mixes
- Vinegar
- Olive or canola oil (these will be used sparingly)
- Vegetable oil spray, purchased or homemade by filling a spray bottle 2/3 with water and the remaining 1/3 with olive or canola oil. Shake well before each use.
- Assorted spices (Italian, Cajun, garlic powder, rosemary, thyme, basil, etc)

Again, if you purchase canned vegetables either purchase the lower sodium variety versions or rinse well to remove salt in the regular varieties.

In the refrigerator/freezer

- Low fat yogurt (you can buy the fruit-flavored versions, but you can save money by buying large containers of plain yogurt and adding fruit later)

- Vegetable rich, low fat, lower sodium frozen dinners

- Stir-fry vegetables (to save money, buy the versions without sauce; add low sodium soy sauce later)

- Whole wheat bread or tortillas (you can freeze these items – use heavy freezer bags, expelling as much air from them as possible. They should last 2-4 weeks)

- Frozen orange juice concentrates (go for the variety with the pulp for a little fiber)

If you keep your kitchen well-stocked with the staple items above, then you can just add a few other items to make a complete, healthy meal on the days when you don't have a lot of time to cook. The following are some examples of quick meals you can have for breakfast:

- Fruit smoothie: Mix together 1 cup of frozen berries or bananas, 1 cup of skim or 1% milk and 1/2 c. of vanilla-flavored yogurt, 1 TBSP honey and blend until smooth. As a variation, you can also use a scoop of vanilla or chocolate flavored protein powder as a substitute for the yogurt. If you love milkshakes, you will be very fond of smoothies!

- Oatmeal with brown sugar and cinnamon to taste; slice a baked apple and stir in for a great-tasting variation.

- Fruit flavored yogurt with ¼ cup of almonds or walnuts

- Medium whole wheat pancakes with small amount of syrup and butter to taste; ½ cup of mixed berries

- 1 cup of high-fiber cold cereal with 1 cup of 1% or skimmed milk and ½ banana

Some examples of a quick lunch or dinner are as follows:

- Vegetable soup: Simply add any fresh vegetables such as peas, carrots, potatoes, or corn to canned vegetables or chicken broth and cook over medium heat until the vegetables are tender

- Chili: Mix together canned tomatoes, black beans or kidney beans with some chopped peppers and onions. Add spices like chili powder, dried onion, cumin, cayenne pepper, and garlic to your taste.

- Omelets or scrambles: You can use eggs, low fat cheese, and some leftover vegetables to make a deliciously different dinner.

- Mini-pizza: Cover a whole wheat bagel with some chunky spaghetti sauce. Top with the vegetables of your choice, such as mushrooms, artichokes, peppers, or onions. Finish with part-skim mozzarella cheese and melt under the broiler.

- Burritos: Fill a whole wheat tortilla with cooked onions, peppers, canned chicken, low fat cheese, and salsa. You can also use black beans instead of chicken for a vegetarian variation.

Some quick snack ideas are:

- High fiber fruits such as apples, pears, and berries
- 3 cups of air popped popcorn with 2 tbsp of Parmesan cheese
- 1 protein energy bar (at least 7 grams of protein, plus 2 grams of fiber, and 150 calories or less).
- 1 oz container of fat-free fruit yogurt
- 1 cup strawberries with 1/2 c of cottage cheese or low fat Ricotta cheese (you can add a natural sweetener or small amount of sugar substitute)
- Low sodium tomato or vegetable soup
- 1 cup of carrot, red pepper, and celery sticks with 1 oz low fat cheese
- Ginger snaps or animal crackers (3 or 4 cookies maximum)
- Graham crackers (1 cookie)
- Sugar free pudding snacks/cups

From the meal preparation ideas, you hopefully see that the guiding principle is to include fruits or vegetables as often as possible (even snacks). This is the easiest way to ensure that you get the recommended number of servings to achieve your health and weight loss goals. Think of it as a game; how much color can you add to your meals? Brown is bland! Spice things up by adding red, green, purple, and orange to your plate. Here are some more ideas to increase your fruit and vegetable intake:

- Have a piece of fruit with breakfast, like bananas, grapes, or berries
- Eat a large salad for lunch
- Add sliced tomatoes, onions, peppers, or lettuce to sandwiches
- Add at least three vegetables servings to your lunch and two servings to your dinner

The deeper the color of the fruit or vegetable, the more nutrients it can provide, so look for richest, deepest colors available. As passionate as you might be for foods that aren't healthy, you must make your passion for healthy foods even greater.

HEALTHY FOOD PREPARATION

When preparing meals, keep in mind one important point: get rid of the grease! Think about it; if you have ever prepared fried chicken or fish, did you ever pour the grease down the drain? You probably didn't because you knew that the grease would clog the pipes. You would have to either try to remove the clog yourself or incur expensive repair bills if a plumber is needed to do the job.

Think of your body's circulatory system as comprised of a series of pipes, literally known as blood vessels. These vessels are much smaller than the pipes in your house. What do you think eventually happens when you pour that same grease down your throat via the foods you eat? It clogs your pipes!

If the clog is near your heart, blood flow and oxygen is cut off to that muscle, causing a heart attack. If the blockage is in one of the vessels that delivers blood and oxygen to your brain, then a stroke results. Either way, you can cause serious damage. Do your body a favor and limit eating fried foods as much as possible.

You can enjoy the taste of fried food if you opt for "oven frying" food with non-saturated oils such as canola or olive oil. This method makes your food crispy without the extra grease. Some recipes for oven-fried fish and chicken appear in the Recipes section.

Since you will be doing a great service to your body by increasing your fruit and vegetable intake, you don't want to blow it by preparing them with a lot of fat/grease. An alternative way to get great taste is to bake or roast vegetables. Baking vegetables brings out their sweetness and flavor. Other great ways to prepare meals are to grill, broil, boil, steam, poach, or sauté your vegetables. Be sure to add spices, sautéed onions and/or garlic for flavor.

You can also steam your vegetables in low sodium chicken or vegetable broth for flavor. You will soon begin to prefer these methods to frying since they allow you to taste the food instead of the flavor being buried under grease.

In addition, you can adjust your favorite recipes to help you meet your health and weight loss goals. Try the substitutions in the table that follows. You might have to experiment with the amounts so that you can get the same results without excess fat, but the effort will be worth it.

If the recipe calls for...	Then substitute
Regular mayonnaise	Light or fat-free mayonnaise
1 whole egg	2 egg whites
Whole milk	1% milk or skim milk

Sour cream	Non-fat plain yogurt or non-fat sour cream
Regular cheese	Part-skim or 2% milk cheese
Whipping cream in recipes	Evaporated skim milk, chilled
Butter (for browning)	Vegetable oil cooking spray
1 cup of sugar	3/4 cup of sugar
Oil (baking recipes)	For yellow cake recipes, use applesauce or mashed banana in an amount equal to the amount of oil in the recipe. For chocolate cake recipes, use baby food prunes in an amount equal to the amount of oil in the recipe.
Cream soup	Low fat cream soup
Regular bouillon and broth	Low sodium bouillon and broth
Pork (Ham hocks, fat back)	Turkey ham, turkey bacon, smoked turkey wings or necks, skinless chicken thighs
Bacon	Turkey bacon or Canadian bacon
Lard, butter, or other hard fats	Small amounts of vegetable oil, such as canola or olive oil

GUIDELINES FOR EATING OUT

The following are some guidelines to use if you will be eating at a fast food restaurant. If possible, check out the restaurant's Web site before you go since most of them post menu nutritional facts on their sites. You can then make wise decisions as to what to order.

- Order sandwiches with whole grain bread instead of white if available.
- Avoid deep fried fish or chicken sandwiches. They sound healthy, but often have more fat than the small hamburgers.
- Avoid any sandwiches with multiple buns or hamburger patties.
- If healthier options aren't available, order the smallest size available or the junior size of hamburgers, fries, etc.
- Order sandwiches without mayonnaise or sauce. Add lowfat mayonnaise, ketchup, or mustard later.
- Order a tomato-based soup, corn on the cob, baked potato with chili, or salad as a side item instead of French fries or onion rings.
- Limit soft drinks. Go for water, small juice, or 1% milk.
- Opt for extra vegetables on pizza rather than extra meat; Avoid bread appetizers.

If you are accustomed to eating out in sit down restaurants frequently, you will save money just by decreasing those visits to once a week or every other week. The following guidelines will keep your nutritional goals on track during restaurant visits:

- Ask for a To Go box or doggie bag when you place your order. Place half of your food in the container when it arrives. Since restaurants typically provide *two to three times* a normal serving size, you will save your waistline and have an additional meal for later when you practice this strategy.
- Try ordering one entrée and splitting it with a friend. Just ask the waitperson for an extra plate. The restaurant might charge you for the plate, but it will still be less than the entrée.
- Choose a vegetable-rich main dish, like a vegetable stir-fry or dinner salad.
- If ordering salads, ask for your salad dressings on the side. Dip your fork into the dressing and stab the greens to get the taste of the dressing but without the excess.
- Order main dishes that come with a side of vegetables. You can also ask for a side of vegetables instead of fries and rice.
- Avoid dishes described as rich, creamy, fried, or crispy. Choose dishes described as grilled, tomato-based, cooked in broth, au jus (or in its own juice).

Small Steps Action Plan - Healthy Food and Preparation

Place a checkmark next to the actions you are willing to take to practice healthy food selection and preparation. Review this list once a week to be sure you are following through on your decision.

❑ I make fruits and vegetables the cornerstone of my diet.

❑ I make water my preferred fluid source.

❑ I keep my cabinets and pantry well stocked with healthy staple items.

❑ I pick at least one or two items from the suggested quick meals to try when time is limited.

❑ I prepare meals by grilling, broiling, boiling, steaming, poaching, or sautéing, not frying.

❑ With rich recipes that I love, I adjust them using the recipe substitution guidelines in the chapter.

❑ I will practice wise menu selection strategies if eating at fast food restaurants or sit down restaurants.

Chapter 6: Move It and Lose It

"Lack of activity destroys the good condition of every human being, while movement and methodical physical exercise save it and preserve it."

— Plato, Ancient Philosopher

The acknowledged "Father of medicine," Hippocrates, noted that the body becomes healthier, well developed, and ages more slowly when exercised in moderation. He also stated that the body becomes liable to disease and ages quickly if unused. His advice is an illustration of the old adage "Use it or lose it." In this chapter, you will learn about effective ways to *move it and lose it*, not your mobility but your excess weight.

Why is exercise important? Think of your excess fat as like gas in a tank—it is stored energy. Just like a car can only burn gas when turned on, your body can only burn fat when the engines (muscles) of your body are engaged.

Your body was created to move. It is supposed to feel good. When you were a child, did anyone have to force you to play or go outside for recess? Of course not!

Moving your body today should be viewed in the same way—as an opportunity to play.

So start playing again!

Thinking of exercise as play and using your imagination to make it fun might be a new concept for you but it's important for you to succeed. Remember when you read that the Limbic system part of our brain loves pleasure? One way you can associate pleasure to your exercise program is to start with an activity that you love or at least, don't dread. Every extra movement done with purpose counts—even common activities like gardening or cleaning up your house.

Try this activity. Think about how many pounds you want to lose. Each pound represents stored energy that you want to burn. Think about some activities around your house that you need to do, then make a list and assign a pound amount to them. For example:

- Washing my car by hand – ½ pound

- Washing the dishes by hand – ¼ pound

- Mopping my kitchen floor – 1 pound

- Weeding my garden – 1 pound

- Cleaning out my closet – ½ pound

Next, practice what I call the 15-minute solution.

The 15-minute solution means that for 15 minutes in the morning and 15 minutes in the evening, you set aside time to perform one of the activities on your list or to pick up after yourself. If the activity you pick is cleaning out your closet, then decide ahead of time which section you can realistically finish within 15 minutes. You might spend your 15 minutes just organizing the top shelf if your closet is cluttered!

As you complete each task, imagine yourself actually losing the amount of weight you've assigned to it. Not only will you complete tasks you might have been putting off but you will also start to see how even ordinary physical activity will help you accomplish your health goal. The real secret to making this activity work for you is to turbo charge your movements. View getting healthy and fit as an exciting game.

So instead of housecleaning, do power house cleaning, instead of just vacuuming, make it super vacuuming. Do the chores that you would have done anyway with more energy and enthusiasm. The 15-minute solution helps you do them more often so that you will have a cleaner house along with a fitter body.

Even small amounts of extra activity add up. I found out this the hard way. I figured out that I had gained nearly 100 pounds by overeating 50 calories per day consistently over 20 years. If I had instead exercised that 50 calories off each day, the weight gain *never would have happened.*

The following are exercises that would have burned the 50 calories:

- 10 minutes of light dancing

- 10 minutes of light cycling

- 15 minutes of light walking

- 5 minutes of jump roping

- 7 minutes of light aerobics class

- 7 minutes of stair climbing

While it didn't take much for me to gain weight, it wouldn't have taken a lot to prevent it either. The power of consistency would have been working for me instead of against me. All it would have required was to expend just a little more energy than I typically did each day.

Engaging in consistent activity is an investment in your future health. In my case, I choose to invest four to five hours per week in exercise. The way I view it, my five hours of exercise each week yields 112 hours (the number of waking hours in a week) of enjoying a healthier, slimmer, more toned, and energetic body. What a return on an investment!

Let's put it another way. If a friend asked you to loan her $5 on Sunday, and promised to pay you back $112 on the upcoming Saturday, would you do it? You bet you would! If that friend continued to offer you the same deal for a month, how much do you think you would have? Well, for your investment of $20, you would have $448 at the end of the month.

If you were offered the same deal for 3 months, your money input would be $60 but the amount you would be paid is $1,344! Amazing, isn't it? Think of not moving your body purposely for the next three months as equivalent to leaving $1,344 on the table, except in this case, it's 1,344 hours.

Convinced that investing in exercise is worth your time? Then let's look at the best ways to redeem that time.

Fun

Use your imagination to make exercise fun. If you are dancing, pretend that you are doing so in front of a live audience on Broadway; if you are walking, pretend that you are racing an imaginary opponent or that you are being timed to reach the next tree or landmark.

Children are great role models when it comes to movement. When they want to move, they get up, jump around, spin, or skip. When they are tired, they sit...but not for long. Take the same attitude.

If you feel restless, then move even if it's just to stand up and stretch or pace. It doesn't seem like much, but it adds up. You subtly communicate to your body that you are now an active person rather than a sedentary one and you'll burn calories more efficiently.

The following fun activities allow you to move your body in less formal ways:

- Take a day to play with your children, if you have them. Get out into the sunshine and breathe in some fresh air. Toss the ball with them, play hide-and-seek or a game of hopscotch. Maybe you can challenge them to a duel with water guns on a hot day, or get them to teach you how to skate. If you do not have children, borrow the neighbor's children for a while! Go back to childhood to get out of your rut.

- Speaking of childhood, did you have a special sports goal that you wanted to achieve? Did you want to be a dancer, ball player, or karate master? Get creative and ask yourself if you can give yourself a taste of that dream as an adult right now. You might be able to find a class that offers adult lessons in ballet or tap dance at a YWCA. You might even find an adult baseball league that plays in your local park. Do you see some possibilities here? Make movement, any kind of movement, a vital part of your day.

- Watch a dance movie like *Grease*, *West Side Story*, or *Footloose*. Whenever the characters dance, you get up and dance, too.

- Get a hula hoop at a dollar or discount store. It's not that different from the hip movements you learn in a belly dancing class.

Also use your creativity to think of movement "games" you can play. Try the games that follow or make up your own:

- **Racewalking championship**

  When you are out walking, pick someone who is walking several feet ahead of you and pretend that you are in a race with him/her. If you are able to pass the person, you win. But even if you "lose" the race, you still win in the health arena.

- **Climb the Matterhorn**

  Whenever you see a staircase, tell yourself, "Time to climb the Matterhorn (or Mount Everest or any other mountain name you want to use)" and then climb those stairs. It is challenging, but if you make yourself feel like "Rocky" when you reach the top, you will find yourself actually looking for stairs to climb. I do.

- **The Supermodel walk**

  Pretend that you are a supermodel and walk fast, with your head held high, and exaggerate the sway of your hips, with one foot slightly crossing in front of the other as you walk. Pretend that you are on a runway in Paris modeling the latest fashions or that you are on your way to a magazine photo shoot and you must hurry.

- **Grocery relay**

  Instead of loading yourself down with groceries, take in only two bags at a time, maximum. Walk as fast as you can to take them into the house, and then run back to the car to get the next two. This can be especially fun if you have children, because they can stand by the car and relay the bags to you. Believe me, they will enjoy watching Mom or Dad run!

Function

Functional exercises help increase your endurance. Endurance is staying power, or the ability to sustain an activity for extended periods of time. Exercise also improves your circulation and cardiovascular health. Finally, it produces feel good chemicals like endorphins and serotonin, which as explained before, leave you with a sense of well-being and calm alertness.

What are some of the best exercises for increasing energy and endurance? Exercises that involve the large muscle groups in the body such as those of the legs and backside are best. These exercises are aerobic dancing, jogging or running, walking, rebounding, bicycling or stationary biking, jumping rope, cross-country skiing, and stair climbing or elliptical training.

All of these exercises help increase energy and endurance because they are aerobic activities, which means *with oxygen*. The exercises are challenging, but you perform them at a comfortable level so that there's plenty of oxygen supplied to your body during the activity.

Before you start an exercise program, please consult your physician to be sure that you do not have any conditions that affect your ability to exercise. This is especially important if you are over 35 or severely overweight.

Types of function activities

Let's take a closer look at function activities. With each exercise, the number of calories burned is listed. The heavier you are, the more calories you will burn with exercise. A great online resource for assessing the number of calories burned with exercise is http://www.caloriecontrol.org. Look for the exercise calculators on this Web site.

One word of advice: when evaluating exercises, the number of calories you burn should not be the deciding factor. What matters is choosing an exercise that you know you will be consistent in performing. After all, what good does it do to jump rope when you can only do it two or three sessions before wanting to quit? It would be better if you pick walking if you think that you'll be able to do it five times a week for three months (60 sessions).

The exercises that are less strenuous are listed first:

- Walking is the easiest exercise to do because it doesn't require special equipment and is gentle enough for you to do every day. It also tones all of your lower body muscles but without stress on your hips, knees, and back.

If walking will be your primary exercise for weight loss, then your pace needs to be comfortable, but also challenging. You must exercise at a pace that stretches your body slightly beyond its limits. Only then will it adapt by improving your cardiovascular health and by dropping excess pounds.

- Swimming is a great exercise that tones most of the muscles in the body, not just the muscles of the lower body. Because it is a non-weight bearing activity, the exercise is advantageous to the overweight or physically challenged. The water provides buoyancy and does not stress joints. It is recommended that you start by swimming 100 yards three times a week, then eventually work up to 550 yards on most days of the week.

- Mini trampoline/rebounding is a fun activity that takes you back to childhood and is a good alternative for people who need to avoid high impact activities, such as jogging. More than merely jumping up and down, many rebounding routines allow you to perform strength training as well as aerobic activities. You can either create your own routines or check out some of the rebounding exercise videos at the Collage Video Web site at http://www.collagevideo.com.

- Aerobic dancing is one of the more entertaining forms of exercise. You can participate in formal classes at a gym, purchase exercise DVDs for use at home, or even put on some music from your younger days and dance. Lively Christian music works great too! You can find exercise DVDs at discount stores like Walmart or you can go to the Collage Video Web site to compare videos and order online.

  You can add variety to your routine by trying programs based on Latin dance, ballet, jazz, or even kickboxing. Spiritual dance is also a great way to exercise and worship at the same time.

  In addition to improving your energy and endurance, aerobic dancing tones your stomach muscles, hips, thighs, and backside.

- Bicycling and stationary bicycling can take you back to those carefree days of childhood. Unlike some other exercises, the bike helps support your weight, so there is less stress on your bones and joints. This exercise tones all of your lower body muscles, including your backside, thighs, and calves.

If you choose to use outdoor biking as a primary exercise, you will need to outfit yourself with the proper safety equipment, such as a helmet. You will also need to wear weather appropriate and reflective clothing, especially if you plan to bike during evening hours when drivers on the road may have difficulty seeing you.

Stationary bicycling gives you some of the same benefits as outdoor biking. The only drawback for doing this is that some find it repetitive. However, you can always watch TV, play music, or mount a bookstand so that you can read to occupy your mind.

If you are the more social type, you might even consider joining a spinning class at a local health club if within your budget. Spinning classes put a different spin on stationary biking in that the mind/body connection is explored. The instructor varies the workout speed and intensity and may ask participants to imagine different scenarios as they bike, such as racing in the *Tour de France* or climbing hills.

- For an exercise that increases endurance and energy, running is hard to beat. Jogging is simply a slower version of running. This activity tones the thighs, backside, calves, and also the stomach muscles to a lesser extent. The only caution with running is that it is not recommended for those who have existing knee and hip problems. If done in excess, it may also contribute to future joint or knee problems.

For larger-breasted women, jogging can be uncomfortable without the proper breast support. If you are larger breasted, I highly recommend a sports bra that is manufactured by Enell. To learn more, visit their Web site at http://www.enell.com.

For beginners, I do not recommend jogging unless you are already moderately fit. Start with walking first. As your leg strength and lung capacity increase, you can accelerate to jogging. Otherwise, you risk injury and then you would not be able to exercise at all.

- If you like exercising with machines, a step machine or an elliptical trainer might be ideal for you. This exercise defines the lower body muscles. But like running, this exercise can be challenging for beginners so begin slowly and gradually increase your time on the machine.

- Finally, there's the jump rope, which is one of my favorite exercises. In addition to toning the lower body muscles, this activity burns a lot of calories in a short period of time. Jumping rope is also an inexpensive activity.

You want to use one of the vinyl or rubber jump ropes available. For comfort, wear a good sport bra and a supportive cross-training shoe or dance sneaker.

At first, try alternate jumping and walking in between to catch your breath. As your endurance increases, you will jump more and walk less. Try jumping for 16 turns, then walk for 20 seconds to catch your breath. Alternate this pace until your time is up.

The best surface on which to practice jump roping is a suspended wooden floor. When you jump, pretend that you have a ceiling barrier that is about 2 inches over your head. Keeping your jumping height low should help prevent extra stress on your knees and other joints.

Since your primary goal is to lose weight, I recommend that you perform a function activity at least 5 times per week, which gives you two rest days per week.

Pick two activities from the list above or select another aerobic activity with which to alternate. That way, you get the benefits of cross training, which allows you to work different muscle groups and obtain faster results.

Start slow by setting a goal of 15 minutes each session if you haven't been exercising. Add 5 minutes per week until you are exercising for a minimum of 45 minutes each time. If you find yourself pressed for time, try doing two sessions of just over 20 minutes each on exercise days or even three 15 minutes sessions. You will get the same benefits.

Whatever exercise you choose, consistency is the key to getting results. With consistency, your body will become a fat-burning machine instead of a fat storing one. So resolve to stick with it, gradually increasing your minutes as you grow strong and fit. With consistent effort, you will soon experience new levels of energy and vitality, not to mention feeling more confident.

Form

If you like instant gratification, strength training is the ideal activity for you. Strength is the ability to exert force against resistance. In everyday life, you need strength to carry grocery bags, move furniture, or lift a child. One of the other benefits of strength training is that it allows you to define your muscles, which helps you look better in your clothes.

Most people see increases in strength in a matter of weeks. As you improve with your strength training efforts, you'll also notice increased confidence and your endurance activities will become easier, which can motivate you to continue working out.

Strength training is important because after age 35, we lose ½ pound of muscle per year and gain 1 ½ pound of fat per year. This is detrimental for two reasons: Because fat takes up more room than muscle, we will start to see the infamous "middle-age spread." In addition, muscle burns more calories than fat, so by replacing muscle with fat, we'll burn fewer calories even at rest, resulting in increased weight gain.

If you perform regular strength training, you will lose fat much faster. Your muscles are the engine of your body and as such, they will burn your excess fat—even while you sleep!

Many women don't want to strength train because they are afraid of bulking up when they do. You don't have to worry; the male hormone testosterone governs muscle gain and women have very little of it. Women bodybuilders usually follow strict diets and intense exercise programs involving very heavy weights. Some may even use performance enhancing drugs to gain muscle. Your strength-training program should yield the benefits of adding muscle but without the bulk.

Types of form activities

What are some examples of form activities? Weight training falls into this category, either using dumbbells, resistance bands, or the weight of your own body.

Before you perform any type of strength training exercise, you want to be sure that your muscles are warmed up, which will help you avoid injury. You can perform any kind of rhythmic activity to warm up, such as walking or dancing, for five to ten minutes.

The American College of Sports Medicine (ACSM) recommends that most people complete eight to 12 repetitions of each exercise for maximum results. A repetition is completing the exercise described once in a controlled manner.

After you complete the recommended number of repetitions, rest for a minute or two, and then perform another set. You may perform up to three sets of each exercise.

When you strength train, make your movements smooth. Breathe deeply and evenly, inhaling on the easier part of the exercise, exhaling on the effort. Be sure to extend the muscle through its full range of motion.

Now let's take a look at some of the muscle groups and the types of exercises that can help strengthen them. These exercises use your own body weight for resistance:

- The stomach muscles can be strengthened by exercises such as crunches and sit-ups. Crunches can be performed in a variety of positions to work all sides of the abdominal muscle. These exercises can help you improve your posture and also help you perform better if you participate in sports that require a lot of side-to-side motion, such as swimming and baseball.

Performing crunches: Lie on your back with your knees bent and your feet flat on the floor. Place your hands behind your head. Raise your head and shoulders off of the floor, keeping your lower back in contact with the floor. Keep your elbows back and neck straight as you lift your upper body. Feel the tension in the stomach muscles, then lower your shoulders slowly, and repeat.

To perform a reverse crunch to work your lower abdominal muscles, lie on your back with your legs bent and your feet flat on the floor. Place your hands behind your head. This time, raise your knees up to your stomach, keeping your legs together, and your lower back in contact with the floor. Then, return your legs back to the starting position with your feet on the floor. Repeat.

- Squats and lunges are the best strength training exercises to help build strength in your lower body, because they work your thighs, calves, and backside. You can also perform leg lifts in different positions to work the muscles on the inside and outside of your thighs. The calf muscles are very strong and are attached to the strongest tendon in the body, the Achilles tendon. To keep your calves healthy, simply stand on your tiptoes for eight to twelve repetitions, rest a few seconds, and then repeat.

Performing squats: Keeping your back straight, your head up, and your hands out in front for balance, slowly descend into a seated position, with legs bent at a 90-degree angle. Then push up from your heels to a straight-standing position, keeping your feet on the floor. Depending on your current strength, try doing two sets of 10 to 20 repetitions of each exercise, and increase gradually from there.

• To increase strength in your upper body, you can perform push-ups and pull-ups, which use your own body as resistance, or you can use light three- to five-pound weights. Exercises like the 'biceps curl' work the muscles on the front of the upper arm, while exercises like the 'triceps kickback' work the muscles on the back of the upper arm. The muscles in the lower part of the arm are worked simply by holding the weights. See the Resources section for book recommendations that illustrate strength training exercises.

Performing pushups: Keep your back straight and your palms flat, slightly wider than shoulder width.

Descend slowly, until your chest and hips are inches from the floor. Push up faster than you came down, pause at the top, and repeat.

After your strength training session, it is very important to stretch the muscles that have been worked. Stretching increases blood flow to the muscles, which helps prevent soreness.

Like all exercise programs, start slowly with strength training. It is recommended that strength training be done three days a week on non-consecutive days. Muscles need at least forty-eight hours to rest and repair themselves.

If you choose to strength train for more days, be sure not to work the same muscle groups on consecutive days. For example, if you work the muscles in your upper body on Monday, then work the muscles in your lower body on Tuesday. This gives the muscles in your upper body time to rest. You should be able to work the muscles in your upper body again on Wednesday.

With the unbeatable combination of endurance and strength training, you will find yourself feeling more comfortable in your ability to handle everyday stressful situations. You can also be secure in the knowledge that you are engaging in activities that will benefit you into your golden years.

Flexibility

Your exercise program would not be complete without adding flexibility training to your workout. Flexibility becomes more important as you age, since so many of us lose the ability to move our joints through their fullest range of motion. Just like all of the other exercises, flexibility exercises help make your daily activities easier.

Even now, you might find yourself moving more slowly to get out bed or groaning if you have to pick up a piece of paper off the floor. If you suffer from problems like lower back pain, flexibility training can help to decrease the discomfort.

Most people can safely perform flexibility exercises every day. One of the best times to stretch your body is after you take a warm shower or bath. Take each of your joints through their fullest range of motion.

Try these stretches:

Towel stretch: Stand with your feet shoulder-width apart, holding the ends of a towel in both your hands.

Raise your arms to chest level in front of you. Rotate your arms to the right, back and left, stretching your upper back and shoulders. Repeat this movement five times clockwise, and then reverse the motion counterclockwise. This technique releases tension in the upper back and shoulders.

Forward bend: Stand erect with your legs straight. Bend forward at the waist slowly with knees slightly bent, and touch your toes lightly with your fingers. If you can't touch your toes yet, just go as far as you can. Stand upright again slowly, one vertebrae at a time. Repeat the sequence ten times.

Hold each stretch for thirty to sixty seconds. Strive to stretch just to the point of a slight challenge, not until you feel pain. Be patient with yourself. If you can't stretch as far as you'd like, realize that the more you practice and the more your muscles loosen up, the farther you will be able to stretch.

Patience is a virtue (and fruit of the Holy Spirit) that will serve you well in starting an exercise program Experts estimate that it takes twenty-one days of consistent practice for a new habit to take hold. So resolve to put in the necessary time and give yourself credit for your progress. That way, you will not only enjoy your final destination, but every step you took to get there.

STAYING MOTIVATED

I have long established an exercise habit yet still have days when I don't feel like doing it. On those days, I always tell myself, "I don't wanna, but I'm gonna." Then, I go ahead and do it, striving to complete 10 minutes. By the 10 minute mark, I've usually warmed up and want to continue. Another technique I will use to motivate myself to start is to recall my childhood and how I felt riding a bike or racing someone. Infusing those feelings into my current routine usually helps.

However, if I still don't want to exercise that day after completing 10 minutes, then I don't. I have found it best to listen to your body and respect its strengths and limitations. Some days you will feel like you can climb Mount Everest and other days, you will feel like you can't climb out of bed. Strive to do the best you can with the energy your body has available that particular day and you will reach your fitness goals faster.

Here are some other ways you can motivate yourself:

- Begin an exercise checklist to keep track of your workouts. At the beginning of the week, decide on the activities that you are going to do and check off each one upon completion. You will have a real sense of accomplishment when you view your record at the end of the week.

- Find an accountability partner. This person will serve as a combination coach/role model for you. You want this person to be someone who has already achieved the level of health that you want. Ask that person if he/she would be willing to review your exercise checklists each week to help you stay accountable.

  Again, it is best to choose someone who has already achieved what you want, not someone who is in the same condition as you. If the partner you choose is on the same level, then they might unconsciously sabotage you if they find themselves slipping. It's best not to take the risk.

- Become your own encourager by creating an "inspiration station" box. Just decorate an old shoebox and place scriptures, quotes, poems, song lyrics, or anything that makes you smile or motivated. Whenever you find yourself losing heart with your efforts, go to the "inspiration station" to pump yourself up.

- Add plenty of variety to your workouts. It is especially important that you change your workouts every 2-3 months. That way, you help prevent over training specific muscle groups and weight plateaus. Once you become fit, a good way to stay motivated is to participate in sports challenges, like charity walks or fun runs.

Losing weight and building health is a process. At times, it may feel like you're pushing a boulder up a hill and you wonder if anything you are doing is making a difference. Be assured that every positive action you are taking is not in vain. Many wonderful things are happening, even if you aren't seeing the results yet.

Each day, focus on the action you are taking and the habits you are building. Use a tape measure and measure your upper arms, waist, and hips before you implement your changes. Every two weeks, re-measure yourself in these areas so that you can see the progress you are making.

I advocate this method of gauging your progress regularly instead of using a scale. Regular scales only show your total weight, not how much fat you've lost. Since muscle weighs more than fat, you may see your weight stay the same if you have gained muscle and lost fat. That is why paying attention to how your clothes fit is important; even though muscle weighs more than fat, it takes up less room.

If you must use a scale, then purchase one of the newer models that also measure your body fat percentage. While the numbers aren't absolutes, they can give you a baseline with which to start. You may see the fat percentage numbers drop, even if the total weight number is the same. Since fat loss is your aim, you will see that you are making progress. No matter which type of scale you use, I recommend that you only weigh yourself every other week since frequently watching the scale more often than that can make you crazy.

If you practice the healthy habits recommended, you should consistently lose between 1 - 2 pounds of fat per week, which is a safe rate for weight loss.

One more thing: Realize that your body is in the driver's seat in determining which parts of your body to burn fat from first. God knows the safest way to accomplish this goal since He designed you and knows your total condition. For example, you might want your body to get rid of your belly fat first, but you reduce your breasts! This will not change no matter how many sit ups you do.

Relax and let your body handle the results. It will eventually burn fat from your problem areas, if you keep your focus on implementing healthy habits daily.

When you practice the physical strategies discussed in this chapter, you will reap abundant rewards. You will have clearer thinking, more restful sleep, and more energy. Best of all, you will soon look in the mirror and be pleased with what you see.

You will be amazed at how the effort to get your body back also strengthens you mentally and spiritually. By gaining control in the health arena, you will also grow in character. With a sharpened character, you will accomplish more of God's intended purpose for your life. You can't ask for a better reward than that.

Small Steps Action Plan - Move It and Lose It

Place a checkmark beside the action steps you will take to incorporate physical activity into your life.

As always, review this list once a week.

❑   I adjust my attitude to think of exercise as an opportunity to play.

❑   I use ordinary household activities to incorporate more activity into my life, either by doing them more often or with more enthusiasm.

❑   I perform functional exercises at least five times a week, 15-45 minutes a session.

❑   I incorporate strength training into my routine two to three days per week.

❑   I practice flexibility exercises most days of the week.

❑   I have adopted at least two of the recommended activities to keep myself motivated.

Part 3

Finishing Touches

Chapter 7: Handling Stress and Temptation

"I know God will not give me anything I can't handle. I just wish He didn't trust me so much."

— **Mother Theresa**

When you are attempting to lose weight and build your health, two big obstacles can derail your efforts: stress and temptation. Stress refers to how you deal with pressure in your life and your body's response to it; temptation is an urge to indulge in an action that you know isn't in your best interest. The key to dealing with both is learning how to shift your mindset and those things on which you tend to focus. It all begins with maintaining an attitude of *accountability*.

An attitude of accountability means taking responsibility for the choices you make or have made. It means not blaming others or circumstances for your choices. Here is a personal story to illustrate this concept.

For years, I suffered from dealing with stress by making poor nutritional choices. Deep down I knew that my coping method wasn't working because even though it helped me relax, it caused me to gain weight and played havoc with my blood pressure. In addition, it decreased my energy and negatively impacted my appearance.

However instead of taking steps to discover a better way of coping with the stress in my life, I focused only on the weight and developed an attitude of "It's not my fault"; "It's not my fault that the fast food restaurants I love are practically on my doorstep"; "It's not my fault that I'm not athletic"; and "It's not my fault that vegetables are so hard to prepare." Do you know where that attitude got me? Nowhere! I stayed overweight and stressed out. Nothing changed...until my attitude did.

How did I change? By telling the truth to myself (that my body is a "temple") and by realizing that I alone was accountable for the food I put in my mouth. I alone was responsible for exercising my body. I alone was accountable for preparing nutritious meals for myself and, on the days when I didn't feel like cooking, I was responsible for buying nutritious meals for myself. I wasn't a child any longer and no one was going to make me healthy but me.

Accountability doesn't mean condemnation when you make mistakes. The condemnation I heaped on myself when I was overweight did nothing to change me.

All it did was make me want to eat more to deal with the pain. Instead, I looked at my circumstances and started focusing on how to get from where I was to where I wanted to be.

So let's discuss stress first. You'll see that maintaining an attitude of accountability is a key part of managing stress and gaining peace.

YOUR PEACE RECIPE

The *Serenity Prayer* is often used in 12-step addiction recovery meetings. However, the prayer is only quoted in part. Here is the complete version:

> *God, grant me the serenity to accept the things I cannot change;*
> *Courage to change the things I can; and*
> *The wisdom to know the difference.*
> *Living one day at a time;*
> *enjoying one moment at a time;*
> *Accepting hardship as the pathway to peace.*
> *Taking, as He did, this sinful world as it is, not as I would have it.*
> *Trusting that He will make all things right, if I surrender to His will.*
> *That I may be reasonably happy in this life,*
> *And supremely happy with Him forever in the next.*

Most times we experience stress because we live our lives contrary to these principles. We refuse to accept circumstances that can't be changed, and experience frustration, anger, and resentment. We refuse to change the circumstances we *can* change and experience depression and low self-esteem. These feelings and peace cannot coexist.

Accepting things that cannot be changed

Accepting things that cannot be changed is one of the most challenging principles to implement in the recipe for peace. For starters, most of us believe that accepting something means to approve of it. In fact, one of the definitions of *accept* is to give admittance or approval.

However, for our purposes, we'll use another definition of acceptance: to endure without protest or reaction. This means not allowing events that you cannot change to frustrate you or cause distress.

What things are you not able to change? If you really ponder this, you will find that many things are outside of your control. Some examples of things that cannot be changed include your height, your heritage, the weather, the past, and another adult's behavior.

Were you surprised by that last one? I am sure that every one of us can remember a time when we tried to change another person. I am also certain that it was a frustrating experience. We can never truly alter another person; we can influence them, but we can't change them.

For example, Nancy's husband always forgot her birthday. She tried leaving him messages on his voice mail at work, she marked the date in red on his desk calendar, and she even left him little notes as reminders, all to no avail.

Every birthday, she used to wait in anxious, silent expectation that he was going to surprise her with a wonderful gift, only to be disappointed when he didn't. She would get angry and stay that way for days after, or she would give him the silent treatment. She even tried not giving *him* a gift on his birthday one year, but that didn't work because he didn't care.

So what were Nancy's choices? Well, she decided that she could either continue to be miserable every birthday by trying to get her husband to do something he either couldn't or was unwilling to do, or she could accept that her husband probably wouldn't ever be the type who remembered birthdays. Nancy chose the latter.

She began to buy her own gifts on her birthday and spend part of the evening with her girlfriends. She didn't make her husband feel guilty and she made sure that she enjoyed her birthday to the fullest. Eventually, her husband began to feel left out of her joy and decided he wanted to join in. He bought her a gift one year and has done so every year since then. All of her reminders and cajoling didn't do a thing to change him. She prayed for him but he had to make the choice to change on his own ultimately.

Another item on the "can't be changed" list is the past. Very few of us can claim that we've made it through life thus far without making some mistakes or without experiencing past hurts. Although we can acknowledge that our past has helped shape who we are today, we should not continue to let the past ruin our present.

Have you ever met people who continue to let their pasts define them? For example, Marie grew up without experiencing much affection from her parents. In fact, her mother in particular was hypercritical, constantly demeaning everything she did. Even though Marie now has a family of her own, she still allows herself to become upset at her mother's comments. She gets angry with her mother and dreads her visits.

Marie does not realize that she has become very much like her mother. She is negative, rarely smiles, and criticizes her own daughters for the smallest mistakes. Yet when someone calls attention to her behavior, she uses her negative childhood to rationalize it.

Marie has the same choices that Nancy had: she can either accept her situation or she can choose not to. She can either forgive her mother for not knowing how to show her love, or she can continue to let her past define her, ruining her chances for present peace and a healthy relationship with her own daughters.

Let's pretend that Marie makes the second choice and chooses to let go of the past so that she can move forward. She accepts that her childhood wasn't the best, but it is over. She forgives her mother for the pain that she caused, realizing that forgiveness is not for the person who hurt her, but a gift that she can give herself.

She does not allow her mother's present criticism to upset her. She realizes that her mother may never change. When her mother criticizes her, she evaluates it. If the criticism is unfounded, she dismisses it. If it is valuable, she decides how to use it constructively.

As for her daughters, she determines to focus on praising their accomplishments rather than being critical of their mistakes. She decides to tell her daughters that she loves them, even if saying the words is difficult at first. If Marie implemented these changes, she would be more peaceful and content. She would be able to enjoy her family and her life more.

Acceptance is your choice. You can either hold onto those things you can't change that cause you stress, or you can let go of them in order to move forward and gain peace.

Carefully consider your life and those things that you need to let go. Accepting these circumstances usually won't happen overnight, but the more you let go, the more peace you will experience.

Courage to Change the Things I Can

British clergyman and historian Thomas Fuller once said, "They do not believe that do not live according to their belief." To see what a person really believes, don't listen to their words; look at their life.

What does your life say about what you value? Is it a true reflection? Your outer world reflects your inner values.

For instance, although my inner values said that I believed in having abundant health and energy when I was obese, my life reflected that I believed in instant gratification. Every time I ate, my behavior said that I believed in eating for my tongue and taste buds rather than for the rest of my body.

Although I usually enjoyed eating junk food while eating it, emotionally I never did. Even if I didn't consciously admit it, I knew deep down that my behavior was not for my highest good. Because I knew that, yet acted in a destructive way, I never experienced peace with my eating habits.

When I finally realized that my behavior was not a true reflection of my values, I sought to change it. I told myself that I was willing to eat nutritiously and exercise daily, whether or not I stayed the same size. I knew that the benefits of eating nutritious food and exercising stretched far beyond any weight issues I had. When my behavior aligned with my inner values, I gained peace in that area.

As the prayer says, it takes courage to change those things that we can. What is courage? It means having the strength to persevere and withstand danger and fear. I believe that fear is the main emotion that holds us back from changing those things we can. Usually we disguise our fear by saying that we are just being cautious.

Fear is a healthy emotion that is designed to make us pause and think before taking an action. Yet too many times, we use this healthy emotion to keep us from those things we most want and deserve. This doesn't mean that you can't ever be afraid, but it means that you should be willing to move forward in spite of it.

Changing circumstances you can alter doesn't mean making big changes overnight. You can take small actions that lead you slowly but surely to the place you want to go. That's what this entire book is about, encouraging you to take small steps toward accomplishing your health goals.

Taking control of the things you can change will give you more confidence than you can imagine. You will be assured that no matter what happens, God will help you handle the next thing that comes along.

Wisdom to Know the Difference

I believe that we all have access to wisdom. Now some of you might say "Well, if I'm so wise, then how come I've made so many mistakes?"

To answer that, I'll ask you a question. Have you ever taken an action, regretted it, and then later told yourself, "I knew I shouldn't have done that?" How did you know? Wasn't there some inner knowing that prompted you to take the path that would lead to your highest good, but you chose to go in another direction? That inner knowing was the conscience God created in you, and the lessons you were taught about discerning right from wrong.

One definition of wisdom is "the ability to judge correctly and follow the best course of action, based on knowledge and understanding." But in order to exercise wisdom in your life, you must first slow down and listen to God speaking to you. True wisdom comes from God alone.

Try this exercise. Resolve to spend thirty minutes completely alone once a week. Make sure that you do this in a location free from distractions. Don't read, watch television, or perform any other activity. Simply sit and reflect. This activity is harder than it sounds. We are so accustomed to having others vie for our attention or occupying ourselves in other ways that we do not know what it is like to be truly alone with ourselves and with God.

At first, you might find yourself having distracting thoughts. You might even feel uncomfortable and restless. Before you know it, you've picked up a book or started some other activity. If that happens, do not get frustrated. Simply sit back down and refocus on your thoughts.

The point of this exercise is to get you used to hearing from God. Many executives have tried this simple technique and say that it often helps them to find solutions to problems that they had previously thought unsolvable. They say that this technique also helps them generate more moneymaking ideas for their businesses.

Alternatively, try writing in a journal in the morning. I often use a journal as part of my Morning Prayer time. As I hear from God, I write down what I heard in my spirit so that I can go back and review it as needed.

Remember one final note as you seek to implement these principles into your daily life. Be patient and kind to yourself. If you find yourself slipping back into your old ways of coping, simply acknowledge your mistake and resolve to improve your behavior at the next opportunity. Keep trying. The rewards for succeeding are tremendous.

ADDITIONAL STRESS MANAGEMENT STRATEGIES

In addition to practicing the principles in the Serenity Prayer, try the following additional tips to help you manage stress more effectively:

Health visualization

Visualization is the process of creating mental pictures. It can be used to reinforce goals that you'd like to reach or to refresh your mind. All you need to begin is your own imagination. Try the following three-minute visualization:

Close your eyes. Inhale, and then exhale slowly. See the number ten appear in your mind's eye, then watch it fade away. Inhale, and then exhale slowly. Then, see the number nine appear, and then slowly fade away. With each number, feel yourself becoming more relaxed. Continue inhaling and exhaling slowly, continuing the countdown from eight to one. Now, the movie is ready to start.

In your mind's eye, scan all of your muscles. Start at the top of your head and work downward, noticing any areas of muscle tension. Imagine golden light infusing each muscle, bringing energy and vitality into it. If a particular muscle feels tense, see the golden light infusing the muscle, warming it, coaxing it into relaxation. After the light has done its job, move on to the next muscle. Repeat the process with any tense muscles you encounter during your scan.

When you have finished your scan, simply inhale and exhale slowly. Visualize the number one in your mind, and then watch the number fade. Inhale and exhale slowly. The number two appears and fades. Continue counting up until you reach ten. After the ten fades, open your eyes and enjoy the feeling of relaxation you have created in your body.

Progressive Relaxation

Progressive relaxation is the granddaddy of all relaxation exercises. To begin, you need to find a quiet place to sit, free from distractions. Assume a comfortable position. You will start at the top of your head, first tensing a muscle group, and then relaxing it completely.

Close your eyes. Inhale and exhale slowly about twenty times, keeping your breath calm and even. Now, tense the muscles in your face, holding the tension for three seconds. Release the tension and relax. Tense the muscles in your neck and shoulders. Hold the tension for three seconds. Release the tension and relax.

Squeeze both fists and tense your arm muscles. Hold for three seconds. Release the tension and relax. Tense your abdominal muscles. Hold for three seconds. Release the tension and relax. Squeeze your buttocks. Hold for three seconds. Release the tension and relax. Tense your leg muscles by pushing your feet firmly onto the floor. Hold for three seconds. Release the tension and relax.

Take a couple of deep, cleansing breaths, noticing the increased feeling of relaxation you have created in your body. Now, reverse the cycle by tensing the muscles of your feet, working your way back up to your face muscles. Again, after you finish, take a few minutes to scan your body and to release any tension that remains.

Aromatherapy

Aromatherapy is the practice of using scents that God created to improve your moods. Studies have shown that just the simple act of inhaling certain scents can make you more alert or induce relaxation. You can normally find aromatic scents in bath and body shops or in some health food stores.

You can put aromatherapy to work for you at home or at work. At home, you can use a scent diffuser. At work, you can use a clean handkerchief to inhale mood-enhancing scents by just dabbing one or two drops of oils on a handkerchief. Let's look at a few aromatic oils and the ways that they can change your mood.

Lavender

Lavender blossoms have a clean, fresh smell. In Europe, physicians recommend using lavender scents to help patients with mood swings, insomnia, and irritability. They also say that it helps contribute to their patient's physical and emotional well being.

Ylang-ylang

Ylang-ylang is sweet and subtle. The scent is simultaneously relaxing and stimulating. Ylang-ylang is frequently used in aromatic candles and bath scents.

Orange

Most of us are familiar with the zesty, refreshing smell of fresh oranges. Orange oil is thought to have a revitalizing and energizing effect on the body. This oil also helps create a calm, alert, positive outlook. Orange oil is especially effective for use in winter months, combating feelings of depression that some experience during those months due to decreased exposure to sunlight.

Lemon

The scent of lemon is often used in cleaning products to bring a bright, clean scent to households. Lemon oil uplifts the body and the mind. Like the scent of oranges, it is thought to inspire calm alertness and mental clarity, and can help decrease feelings of anxiety.

Diaphragmatic breathing

Breath is life. We can live a few days without water, over forty days without food, but only four minutes without air. When you increase the air in your body by practicing regular deep breathing, you bring life to your cells.

This deep belly breathing exercise is a great tool that can relax and invigorate you at the same time. Each action is a multiple of seven:

- Inhale deeply for a count of seven seconds.
- Hold that breath for a count of 14 seconds.
- Exhale completely for a count of 21 seconds.

Repeat this exercise seven times. A good time to practice this activity is before each meal to ensure that you are in a calm, relaxed state when you eat.

HANDLE TEMPTATIONS

To successfully handle temptations, you must first become aware of two things: the mental pictures you create and the meaning you assign to those pictures. The following is a process for handling temptation, which I call the three 'R's:

1. **Recognize the temptation.** When faced with temptation, pay attention to the mental pictures flashing in your mind. If you are being tempted by the thought of chocolate chip cookies, for instance, replace the mental picture you have of them with something outrageous, say a pink elephant.

Also, you will need to change what chocolate chip cookies mean to you. Right now when you think of them they might mean comfort or security. However if you have a tendency to binge on them, you would need to focus on the feelings you get *after* the binge, like depression or feeling out of control.

When you succeed in making the unpleasant feelings associated with a temptation more real to you than the pleasure, you probably will not crave the food as intensely.

2. **Remove yourself from the temptation.** Don't try to be a hero and prove how strong you are by keeping temptation in front of your eyes. Instead, change your environment by either removing yourself or removing the tempting item from your sight. Ideally, you could avoid the cookie aisle altogether!

One of the best ways to avoid temptation is to avoid bringing destructive foods into your home. If you know that a bag of cookies has never lasted more than 24 hours in your house, then face reality. Either don't buy them or buy a single serving snack pack so that your portions are automatically controlled. Snack packs do cost more proportionally but they can be a good alternative if you want a taste of your favorite goodie items but without the temptation that larger bags or boxes can bring.

3. **Seek Reinforcements.** Ask God to reveal the true reasons you want to overeat. Whatever it turns out to be, He can help you face it and overcome it.

Keep the following promise in mind:

> "No temptation has overtaken you except such as is common to man; but God is faithful, who will not allow you to be tempted beyond what you are able, but with the temptation will also make the way of escape, that you may be able to bear it."
>
> - 1 Corinthians 10:13

Overcoming the obstacles described in this chapter takes resolve. But if you monitor your thoughts to ensure that they support your goals and use the techniques described to conquer stress, and fight temptation, then you can be sure of successfully reaching your health goals with laser-like precision.

Small Steps Action Plan - Handling Stress and Temptation

Place a checkmark beside the steps you will take to handle stress and temptation in your daily life.

❏   I maintain an attitude of accountability.

❏   I practice the principles in the Serenity Prayer, accepting things I can't change and changing the things I can (with God's help).

❏   I use the health visualization regularly.

❏   I perform diaphragmatic breathing exercises for relaxation.

❏   I use aromatherapy to uplift my moods or to rejuvenate myself.

❏   I use progressive relaxation exercises to release tension from my body.

❏   I practice the three R's to help me handle temptations.

Chapter 8: Good Health in Action

"Look to your health; and if you have it, praise God, and value it next to a good conscience; for health is the second blessing that we mortals are capable of; a blessing that money cannot buy.

– Izaak Walton, Author

This summary chapter gives you a 'day in the life' perspective of someone who implements the habits suggested in the book on a daily basis. Use them as a guideline to help you accomplish your own health vision.

Since these guidelines are already written as steps, this chapter will not have a 'small steps' checklist for you to complete.

1. Start the day with praise. Spend at least 15 minutes with God, thanking Him for the new day and asking for his wisdom to help you make wise health choices. Ask for His protection and provision.

2. Drink 2 glasses of water (this should be your preferred fluid source). After fasting for 6-8 hours during your sleep, you're bound to be a little dehydrated so use think of the water you drink as a way to "grease" your joints.

3. Eat a balanced breakfast. According to a National Weight Control Registry survey, people who eat breakfast tend to be slimmer than people who do not.

4. Exercise (play) for 45 minutes or break it up into smaller chunks throughout your day (5 minutes, 10 minutes, 15 minutes, etc). Your goal is to accumulate 45 minutes each day, 5 days a week. If you haven't been exercising, then start with 15 minutes of activity and work your way up.

5. Start your praise journal. Write seven things in your journal for which you are grateful. Keeping an attitude of gratitude will help lower your stress level and increase feelings of contentment. Also God will empower you to do great things when you praise Him faithfully.

6. Eat your morning snack. Fruits or vegetables should be your primary snacks, although you can substitute the snacks suggested in chapter five as desired.

7. Eat a properly balanced lunch. Be sure to practice appropriate portion control. Taking a brief walk after lunch will help you digest your food better and also help you handle stressful days with grace.

8. Eat your afternoon snack 2-3 hours after lunch using the same guidelines as the morning snack.

9. Eat a properly balanced dinner, practicing appropriate portion control. One common

problem is eating with control all day but binging at night. A way to prevent this is to drink two glasses of water first, which ensures that you don't consume calories when you are really thirsty.

If you haven't gotten your desired amount of exercise for the day, then you can make it up by taking a walk after dinner.

10. Be sure to go to bed at a time that ensures you get 6-8 hours of sleep. The amount depends on how much sleep you need (some people need more while others need less sleep).

Chapter 9: I've Taken it Back; Now What?

"I know God will not give me anything I can't handle. I just wish He didn't trust me so much."

— Mother Theresa

You've reached your weight loss goal. You look great and you feel even better. What should you do now? Celebrate! You deserve it. Be sure to give yourself a reward for your accomplishments, like purchasing a new outfit, jewelry, scheduling a massage, mini-makeover, or even going on a mini-vacation.

In the midst of your celebration, realize that you might need a period of adjustment to get used to the "new you." I didn't consider this when I embarked upon my own weight loss and was unprepared for it. A few months after achieving my weight loss goal, I had the experience of being pleasantly startled by my own face in the mirror.

I had just awakened and went into the bathroom to wash my face, just like always. But when I looked in the mirror, it was like I was seeing someone new. Without thinking, I blurted out, "Where have *you* been?"

As I stood there looking at myself, I realized that for the first time in a long time, I was looking at the face of the girl who used to be me before I gained weight. She had a heart-shaped face, defined cheekbones, and a sharp chin. While I had a few fine lines under my eyes that weren't there when I was younger, it was the same face otherwise.

I have also had other bodily changes to which I've adjusted: not feeling my thighs rub together when I walk, not having parts "jiggle" when I move, being able to see my muscles, and being able to run. These are all good things, but they did seem odd when I first noticed them. It's funny how when you gain weight, you don't realize the simple things that you sacrifice.

If you have lost a considerable amount of weight, especially after being obese for a long time, you might need time to adjust to walking around in an average-sized body. Many people insist on continuing to wear their plus-sized clothes even after they no longer need them. Somehow their mental picture of themselves hasn't caught up with reality.

Avoid this by ensuring that you wear clothes that are appropriate to your new trimmer size. Create a 'clothes retirement drawer': go through your closet and identify clothes that you can't wear any longer. Place those clothes in the retirement drawer. When you have a sufficient 'inventory' donate those clothes to a charity that accepts used clothing donations such as *Goodwill Industries* or the *Salvation Army*. Since these donations are deductible, you can save money on your taxes plus help another person who needs them.

HANDLING POTENTIAL LETDOWNS

Another potential issue with which you may have to deal in losing weight is disappointment. If you're like me, you've received compliments from others about your weight loss, but no one rolled out the red carpet for you. In fact, some people close to you may even resent your success. You might wonder for a moment if the effort was actually worth it.

It was! Remind yourself that you didn't do this to receive applause from man; you did it to glorify God, to improve the quality of your life, and to start treating your body as the valuable resource it is.

It is not uncommon to think, "Is this all there is?" after losing weight. Most of us fantasized about how our lives would change as a result of losing weight. Some of these expectations might have been realistic ones, like fitting into a smaller clothing size. A few of them might have been unrealistic, like expecting your marriage to become more exciting just because your body is a small size.

For example, let's say that you imagined that when you lost weight, your husband was going to begin taking you out to restaurants, plays, or whisk you off to some really exotic destination. While he has complimented you on your improved health and appearance, your daily life together has actually remained pretty much the same. You feel disappointed.

It's not your fault; you're experiencing a letdown because the world promotes weight loss as the answer to total life change. They always show pictures of the unhappy person lounging in front of the television, but the newly fit person strolling on the beach at sunset, hand-in-hand with the one they love.

What they fail to explain is that losing weight alone will not give you the improved life you seek. Nevertheless, it will certainly improve your health, give you a more pleasing appearance, and make it easier to complete your daily tasks. It will give you energy to *create* the life you want. Otherwise, you will experience the same results that you did before you lost weight. The only difference is that you will be experiencing them from inside a smaller package.

Revisit your expectations. What did you expect would happen when you lost weight that hasn't occurred? These expectations will give you a clue as to what you are really hungering for in your life.

Let's revisit the above marriage example. Your expectation was that your relationship with your husband would be more exciting when you lost weight. The reality is that your relationship is virtually the same. While weight loss alone won't help you achieve this goal, you can work on changing your reality so that it will more closely match your expectation.

You should think of ideas that will help you add more spice to your marriage. Can you take walks together in a local park? Can you take dance lessons together? You want to get creative to help yourself achieve those things you dreamed about at the beginning of your weight loss journey.

Your goal is to acquire a life of balance. Take a look at the categories below and think about the expectations you had regarding how shedding pounds would change these areas. In hindsight, were these expectations realistic? For example, if you expected that you would be discovered by a Hollywood agent and cast as the lead in his next film when you lost weight, then that was probably not realistic.

If your expectations were realistic and achievable according to God's will for your life, then write down your current reality and then how you can change it to match your desire. Here are some of the following areas in your life you might evaluate:

- Family and relationships
- Finances
- Career
- Social life
- Education and training
- Recreation and leisure

Do note that if these expectations involve how other people would change, then those would fall into the unrealistic category. You can only control your own choices; while you can suggest choices to other adults, you cannot make their decisions.

You may not be able to achieve 100% of your expectations but you can move closer to them than before your weight loss. The more content that you are with your life, the more likely it is that you will continue to do the tasks necessary to maintain your weight loss and guard your health.

DON'T GIVE IT BACK

To help you maintain your weight loss and enjoy good health for a lifetime, you will need to adopt some principles to reinforce your new lifestyle. You especially do not want to fall into the same trap as I did—resting on your laurels too long.

Of course to be fair, some aspects of that were unavoidable. For one thing, after losing my first 70 pounds, I had an accident. I fell down some steps and twisted my left knee and ankle. I had knee surgery, and had to have physical therapy to return my knee to full function. The problem was that I knew I had about 20 more pounds I needed to lose, but was no longer motivated to tackle them.

So I maintained my loss for 1 1/2 years. I didn't gain anything, but I didn't lose any more. The truth was that I was scared; I had once said that if I could finally solve my weight problem, which had defeated me for 20 years, I could do anything. What if I was wrong? At least with the weight on, I had an excuse not to go for some of the goals I really wanted to accomplish. With the weight on, I had permission to be less than perfect.

I had to re-evaluate my flawed thought pattern and realize that there is none perfect but God. If He was calling me to a higher standard, then I would be privileged to go forward, trusting that He would equip me with what I need to succeed. Undoubtedly, I was also panicking at the thought of keeping up my good health habits for life. Then I realized that all I had to be concerned about was maintaining them for *today*.

One scripture that brings me great comfort and security is in Psalm 139:5: "You hem me in—behind and before; you have laid your hand upon me. Such knowledge is too wonderful for me, too lofty for me to attain."

This scripture assures me that God redeems my past; He forgives my sins and heals me from any wounds that have occurred from it. So I am hemmed in from *behind.* Also, God has secured my future: in Jeremiah 29:11, he declares that He has plans to give us hope and a future. He cultivates within us the character we need in order to equip us for that future. So, God hems in *before.*

I believe that this security gives Christ followers freedom to enjoy the present in ways others can't imagine. Because God has dealt with our past and is taking care about our future, then we can focus all of our energy and talents on the present.

So the best way to maintain your weight loss is to plan for the anticipated challenges of the day. Start each day by asking God for wisdom in helping you deal with obstacles you may face. For example, you will need to plan your day to make time for exercise and to prepare (or purchase) healthy foods for yourself and your family.

Another part of your plan is anticipating which circumstances might tempt you to fall back into your old health patterns. These circumstances usually correspond to the old Alcoholics Anonymous (AA) adage: Never let yourself get too hungry, angry, lonely, or tired (H.A.L.T).

Here's an example: I recently went grocery shopping when I was hungry and tired. The problem is that *everything* looks good when you are hungry plus you aren't mentally sharp when you are tired. Your body just wants to be fed whether the foods you are choosing are healthy or not.

At that time, I ended up purchasing potato chips. But even though I ate two servings, I soon came to my senses and threw the bag away in the garbage can outside. In the old days, I would have said, "Since I started it, I might as well finish it." Afterwards I would have beaten myself up mentally.

I knew that I had another option; I could minimize the damage by refusing to continue eating the poor food choice. This should always be your goal if you find yourself in the middle of a nutritional meltdown.

The following pages contain more tips that can help you to maintain your weight and health.

Associate with other health-minded individuals

A famous speaker once said that if you want to know where you are going in life, take a look at the people with whom you associate most often. Where they are going is where you will likely go. That's the power of influence.

If most of your friends don't treat their bodies with love and respect then you need to increase your circle to include people who do. You can find such people by participating in a walking group, online fitness discussion groups, nutrition or healthy cooking classes, or gyms. Speak words of encouragement to them by sharing your story and allow yourself to be encouraged by theirs.

Think and speak life to yourself

Start seeing yourself as God sees you. Remember that He calls your body a temple. Earlier I mentioned that the words associated with temple are "beautiful" "sacred" "precious" and "valuable." Now this should not promote an attitude of vanity, but one that has you marveling at the effort it took for God to craft your body. In doing so, you will become more motivated to do what it takes to keep it looking and feeling its best.

Make a list of things that you find attractive about your body. Each day affirm those things by giving yourself at least one compliment. For example, you might say "Wow these earrings really show off my pretty earlobes." It may sound silly, but don't you think it would make you smile?

I met a woman named Valerie in an auto shop recently. We started a conversation and she mentioned that she had lost over 100 pounds. She says that she now starts her day by looking in the mirror and saying out loud: "What am I going to do today? I don't know...guess I'll just have to be beautiful!"

I clapped my hands in delight. Now in mere physical appearance, Valerie didn't look like a movie star but her smile and spirit shown so brightly that her inner beauty surpassed them all. On days when I feel my energy is low I repeat her words to myself and it is amazing how they put extra pep in my step and swing in my stride! Try it and see for yourself.

Daily spiritual refreshment

To picture the importance of receiving daily spiritual refreshment, think of your life as like a tree: Your relationship with God is the root of that tree. Only God can provide the nourishment necessary to keep the tree healthy and flourishing. Communing with Him is as vital to your life as sun and water is to a tree's life.

Your relationship with God also keeps you grounded and stable, no matter what is going on around you. Abiding joy provides a positive perspective on what's really important. Because of my relationship with God I know that no matter what I achieve in my life, I have already accomplished the most important thing: establishing a connection with God through His son Jesus.

Review *Chapter 2: Knowing Your True Source* periodically as a reminder on how to keep your connections with God alive and flourishing. Too often, we fall into a pattern I like to call "branch tending." Each of the roles we have to fulfill (mother, wife, business owner, employee, church worker, etc) is a branch in our lives. Most of us spend so much time tending to these branches that we neglect our roots (relationship with God) and trunk (our physical and emotional health). You might get away with that for a while, but eventually the entire tree suffers because the primary focus is on the wrong part of the tree!

Today shift your focus back to your roots and see your life improve in new, exciting ways!

THE ULTIMATE PRESCRIPTION FOR LIFE

In the bible, the book of Deuteronomy gives the prescription for acquiring abundant life: "… I have set before you life and death, blessing and cursing; therefore choose life, that both you and your descendants may live; that you may love the LORD your God, that you may obey His voice, and that you may cling to Him, for He is your life and the length of your days" (Deuteronomy 30:19-20 NKJV).

God's prescription for life involves just three things:

Love Him, obey His voice, and abide in Him. So the key words are *love*, *obey*, and *abide*.

Spending time with God is a way to show love to Him. In that time, we lay our concerns before Him and receive guidance from Him as to how we should live. As previously recommended, spending time with God is the best way to start your day.

The rest of your day is spent abiding in Him: you consult with Him on the decisions you must make, ask for His provision and protection, and hold praise in your heart for all the goodness and mercy His sends your way.

Each time God speaks to you, obey His voice. Sometimes the things He says don't make sense in human terms but remember that His thoughts are higher than ours and He can see the future while we cannot. Through our obedience to His voice our faith will increase and we will be able to demonstrate what He promised in His word— that our faith would have the ability to move mountains!

So there you have it. You've received the tools to enrich yourself in mind, body, spirit, and even in wallet.

Are you ready to receive everything that God wants you to have? You might think that if you were truly healthy and wealthy that you are somehow robbing others. Nothing could be further from the truth! God is a God of abundance not scarcity. He blesses us so that we can bless others. As an example of God's abundance, all you have to do is look up at the night sky and see how lavishly God decorated it with stars.

You are worth much more than all those stars! So use the prescription in this book to take back your temple, to become a good steward over all the resources God has given you, and to build a legacy of wellness for yourself and your family. Let your light shine before others so that it leads them into abundant life.

Be blessed in health, wealth, and wisdom!

Kim

Small Steps Action Plan - I've Taken it Back...Now What?

Place a checkmark beside the action steps you will take to maintain your good health for life.

As always, review this list once a week.

❑ I give myself a reward for accomplishing my weight/health goal.

❑ I create a 'clothes retirement drawer' for clothes I can wear no longer and donate them to a charity.

❑ I check for unrealistic expectations regarding how my life would change now that I've lost weight.

❑ If my expectations do not match my own reality then I make plans to make them attainable.

❑ I modify the ideal *Take Back Your Temple* day to suit my own lifestyle.

❑ I practice the tips given to help me maintain my weight loss.

❑ I carry out the prescription given so that I can live an abundant life.

My Customized Small Steps Action Plan

Now that you've finished the book, go back to the 'action plan' pages at the end of each chapter. Take a look at each of the small steps you marked, indicating that you can do them. Visualize how you can put these steps into practice and then write your own customized action plan here:

_____

_____

_____

_____

_____

_____

_____

_____

_____

_____

_____

_____

_____

Recipes

Note: Use salt substitutes or salt-free spice blends if you are on a salt-restricted diet. You will find more recipes collections on our website at http://www.takebackyourtemple.com.

Oven Fried Chicken

Ingredients

Vegetable oil spray
4 cups plain corn flakes or bran, crushed

1 tsp. garlic powder

1 teaspoon paprika

1/4 teaspoon salt

Pepper to taste

3 pounds (about 10 pieces) skinless chicken
1 c. of plain nonfat yogurt

Directions

Preheat oven to 375 degrees. Spray flat baking pan with vegetable oil spray. Mix the cereal, garlic powder, paprika, salt, and pepper together in a flat dish or plate.

Rinse chicken and pat dry with paper towels. Dip each piece of chicken in the yogurt, and then coat chicken in cereal crumb mixture. Place chicken in single layer on the baking pan and then spray lightly on all sides with vegetable oil spray.

Bake for 25 minutes, turn chicken over, and then bake for another 20 minutes or until browned and tender. Cooking times vary based on meat thickness.

Oven Fried Fish

Ingredients

Vegetable oil spray

3/4 c. cornmeal
1 tsp. pepper

1 tsp. garlic powder

1 tsp. Cajun spice

1 egg lightly beaten

2 Tbsp. water

2 Tbsp. lemon juice

1 lb. fish fillets (such as whitefish or Alaskan Pollack)

Directions

Preheat oven to 425 degrees. Spray flat baking pan with vegetable oil spray. Mix cornmeal, pepper, garlic powder, and Cajun spice in a large flat dish or plate. Mix egg and water together. Rinse fish and pat dry; sprinkle each filet with lemon juice and dip in egg mixture. Coat the fish with cornmeal mixture and place in pan in single layer. Spray fillets lightly with vegetable oil spray.

Bake for 15 minutes and then turn fish. Bake for another 10 minutes or until fish flakes easily with a fork. Serves four.

Roasted Chicken

Ingredients

Vegetable oil cooking spray

1 TBSP garlic powder

1 TBSP Thyme

1 TBSP Rosemary

1 whole chicken cleaned and rinsed thoroughly

Salt and pepper to taste

Directions

Preheat oven to 375 degrees. Spray a roasting pan with cooking spray. Mix garlic powder, Thyme, Rosemary together. Work your hand under the skin of the chicken breast, being careful not to tear it or pull it off) and rub the spice mixture directly on the breast meat. Also rub some of the spices beneath the skin on the drumsticks.

Spray the chicken lightly with cooking oil spray and sprinkle lightly with salt, pepper, and any remaining spice mixture. Place the chicken in the roasting pan, cover, and bake for 1-1 ½ hours, or until chicken is brown and juices run clear when pierced with a fork. Serves four.

Note: This chicken could be served in pieces or cubed for use in salads, soups, stews, or casseroles.

Sweet Potato Fries

Ingredients

Vegetable oil spray
4 medium sweet potatoes, peeled
1 egg white, lightly beaten
1 Tbsp. Cajun spice

Directions

Preheat oven to 425 degrees. Wash sweet potatoes, and cut into 1/2-inch thick strips. Dry with a paper towel. Set aside. Mix egg white and Cajun spice in a small bowl. Add potato strips to the egg white mixture and coat well. Place in a single layer on a flat baking sheet coated with vegetable oil spray. Bake for about 15 minutes, turn fries and then bake for another 5-10 minutes, or until brown. Serves six.

Smoked Turkey Greens

Ingredients

½ c. red onion

2 cloves of garlic minced

8 cups of turnips greens (cut up - fresh or frozen)

1 Tbsp. apple cider vinegar

3 c. water

1 smoked turkey wing or smoked turkey neck

Dash of salt and pepper to taste

Directions

Place the water, red onion, garlic, and smoked turkey in a large pot and bring to a boil. Reduce to medium heat. Add the turnip greens and cider vinegar. Mix together.

Simmer the greens for approximately 2 hours until tender. When done, season with salt and pepper to taste.

Note: As a meatless variation, substitute 1/2 packet of dry onion soup mix for the turkey wing/neck and red onion.

Fruit Salad

Ingredients

2 cups diced apples (with or without the peel)

2 cups orange wedges

1 banana sliced

1/4 cup diced celery (optional)

1 cup non-fat vanilla yogurt

Directions

Combine apples, oranges, bananas and celery, if desired. Add yogurt and stir until coated. Serve immediately or refrigerate and serve later. Serves four.

Roasted Vegetables

Ingredients

½ pepper (red or green), cut into large pieces

1 large zucchini, sliced

2 large yellow squash, sliced

1 c. sliced mushrooms

½ medium red onion, sliced
5 cloves garlic

2 tbsp. of light balsamic vinaigrette dressing

Directions

Preheat the oven to 375 degrees. Spray a baking pan lightly with olive oil. Place all of the vegetables in the pan and bake for 10 minutes (edges of the vegetables should be lightly browned). Remove the pan from the oven and turn the vegetables over so that the other side of the vegetables is browned. Bake the vegetables for another 5-10 minutes.

Remove the pan from the oven. Place the roasted cloves of garlic in a large bowl. Mash the cloves of garlic. Add the balsamic vinaigrette dressing. Mix the dressing and garlic together. Add the remainder of the vegetables and toss the mixture together. Chill.

Serves four. You can serve as a side dish and use the leftovers in an omelet or as a topping for mini-pizzas (see Chapter 5).

Additional Resources

Health Resources - Books

- *Dr. Ro's Ten Secrets to Livin' Healthy* by Rovenia Brock, PhD., Bantam, 2003

- *Firm for Life* by Anna and Cynthia Benson, Broadway Books, 1998

- *Strong Women Stay Slim* by Miriam Nelson, Bantam, 1999

- *Greater Health God's Way* by Stormie Omartian, 1996 Harvest House Publishers

- *Keeping Fitness Simple* by Porter Shimer, Storey Communications, 1998

Health Resources - Websites

Note: Links are subject to change

- *Cooperative Extension System Offices* (Your county extension office should have the latest information about fruit and vegetables seasons in your area).

  http://www.csrees.usda.gov/Extension/index.html

- *Weight Control Information Network (from the National Institute of Diabetes and Digestive and Kidney Diseases*

  http://win.niddk.nih.gov/

- *Nutrition Education* (From U.S. government Web site on health and nutrition)

  http://www.nutrition.gov/

Wealth Resources

- *Mentored by a Millionaire* by Steven K. Scott, John Wiley and Sons, 2004

- *Your Money Counts* by Howard Dayton, Tyndale House Publishers, 1997

- *Wealth Happens One Day at a Time* by Brooke Stephens, Collins, 2000

- *Start Late, Finish Rich* by David Bach, Broadway, 2005

- *Rich Dad, Poor Dad* by Robert Kiyosaki, Warner Business Books, 2000

- *The Richest Man in Babylon* by George Clason, Signet (reissue edition), 2004

ABOUT THE AUTHOR

Kimberly Floyd has 15 years of health education and training experience through formal nursing practice (as an R.N. for many years) and research on the relationship between nutrition, physical activity, and chronic disease.

She has written training programs for corporate clients, including IBM, U.S. Bank, and The Home Depot. She currently teaches an online course entitled *Goodbye to Shy* which is distributed to 1100 colleges and universities in the United States, Canada, and Australia.

Ms. Floyd's experiences with paying off her debt and shedding pounds prompted her to establish *Take Back Your Temple*, whose title challenges people of faith to take back their health.

In her quest to lose weight, she also discovered how to save money on healthy food. She has combined her weight loss strategies and money-saving strategies into the *MoneyWise Weight Loss* materials.

If you are interested in having Ms. Floyd address your organization or congregation, or for more information about *Take Back Your Temple's* weight management programs and seminars, then please visit us at http://www.takebackyourtemple.com.